AF575216

THE SLENDERNOW DIET

Other books by Dr. Richard Passwater

The Easy No-Flab Diet
Super Calorie & Carbohydrate Counter
Supernutrition
Supernutrition For Healthy Hearts
Selenium As Food & Medicine
Cancer and Its Nutritional Therapies
Guide to Fluorescence Literature, Volumes 1, 2 & 3

THE SLENDERNOW DIET

by Richard Passwater, Ph.D.

St. Martin's Press / Richard Marek
NEW YORK

 For information, write: St. Martin's Press, 175 Fifth Avenue, New York, N.Y. 10010. Manufactured in the United States of America.

Library of Congress Cataloging in Publication Data

Passwater, Richard A.
The slendernow diet.

1. Reducing diets. I. Title.
RM222.2.P353 613.2'5 81-21489
ISBN 0-312-72922-7 AACR2

Design by Stanley S. Drate

10 9 8 7 6 5 4 3 2 1

First Edition

Acknowledgments

I am indebted to the many kind individuals who sent me their success stories. I wish that I could have included more in the book, but even those not included provided valuable data and encouragement to me while preparing the book.

I am also indebted to the Slendernow Neighborhood Clubs of America for "field testing" various aspects of the total Slendernow Diet Program. I am grateful for having the support and encouragement of Allen Skolnick and the technical support of Dave Baucher, Joe Perry, Tom Giles and Keith Kantor. The recipes of Mollie Stein and Pat Raisher will be appreciated by all who use them.

But I am indebted most to the light of my life—my wife, best friend, and partner, all beautifully encased in one lovely person—Barbara. Among many, many important things she does for our boys and me is type and edit my manuscripts.

Introduction

I have used the Slendernow Diet Program personally and in my practice since 1977. It is safe and effective. The Slendernow Diet Program provides weight reduction through controlled, well-balanced nutrition that reduces the number of calories consumed each day, and encourages moderate exercise such as walking briskly. Behavior modification and a maintenance program also are an integral part of the Slendernow Diet Program.

The daily intake of two "Diet Shakes" provides reduced-calories meals, at the same time assuring good nutrition. The daily main meal complements the nutrients contained in the Diet Shakes, and provides a total daily intake of 1200 calories for women and 1500 calories for men. Thus the Slendernow Diet program is designed to forestall hunger, while producing and encouraging a safe rate of weight loss.

Adequate protein is provided for body repair and disease resistance, and adequate carbohydrate is provided to prevent ketosis, fatigue and weakness.

The total nutritional balance of the Slendernow Diet provides it with a good margin of safety that separates it from fad diets.

I find my patients can follow the program without confusion or complicated adjustments to their lifestyle. They enjoy the Diet Shakes and meal menus and are not bothered by hunger. They willingly stay on the Slendernow Diet until they have lost the suggested weight.

At first I questioned the concept of a "meal-in-a-glass." It just doesn't sound like good nutrition until you sit down and analyze it.

The Slendernow Diet provides better total nourishment than most of my patients were getting. Many were overweight but undernourished.

I was curious as to whether the Slendernow Diet could control hunger, so I tried it myself. It did.

I'm sure that many of my colleagues will also recommend the Slendernow Diet if they analyze it and try it themselves.

JOHN H. FORD, JR., M.D.
Miami, Florida

Dr. Ford is Professor at the University of Miami School of Medicine, Department of Obstetrics and Gynecology. His obstetrics and gynecology practice is associated with Jackson Memorial Hospital in Miami, Florida.

Dr. Ford has served as past editor of *Cancer Concepts* and *Miami Medicine.* He has served as past chairman of the Professional Education Committee, Dade County American Cancer Society. Dr. Ford has been appointed to a number of national and local committees dedicated to cancer research and he has published in over a dozen medical books and journals.

Preface

This book describes the details of a complete plan that includes a basic diet, exercise, motivation, behavioral modification, and a maintenance program. Its feature is a protein milkshake, taken twice daily, plus one full meal a day—and exercise. There have, of course, been liquid protein diets, popular a few years ago. These, which were used *instead* of meals, were judged medically unsafe. This is *not* the diet I am recommending here.

My experience with the milkshake, which I will call a "diet shake," for that's what it is, goes back to 1956 when I began serious weight lifting. At that time, I, like thousands of weight lifters and other athletes, used the diet milkshake as a supplement to meals to build muscle.

I continued to use and recommend diet milkshakes to body builders when I was a part-time health club instructor in Wilmington, Delaware, where I was also employed as a full-time chemist. The advantage of being a spa instructor was that it allowed me greater access to the health club for my own training.

Most of the health club clients were interested in weight reduction rather than body building and much of my time was spent helping people lose weight. I saw many fad diets come and go, but it was difficult to interest people in *sound* diets, ones which were safe and effective for everyone. At that time, it had not occurred to me that the protein milkshake could be developed into a meal-in-a-glass.

Credit for that development has been attributed to Lee Causey, owner of a health spa in Jacksonville, Florida. He too was familiar with the use of protein milkshakes for body building and also was involved in helping people lose excess weight as well as build bodies. He was troubled by the fad diets used by some of his health club patrons, and was distressed that they couldn't or wouldn't follow sensible diets. While extolling the excellent nutrition of the protein milkshake, it occurred to Lee that they also would be good as a supplement to the poor diets used in popular weight-loss programs. Lee recognized that while the milkshakes were highly nutritious, they were low in calories. As Lee began implementing his dieting ideas at his health spa, he soon perfected the basic two-milkshakes-a-day-plus-a-meal diet. Without his ideas, this book would not exist.

The first commercialization of this diet concept involved a protein powder product called "Slendernow," produced and first used by Mark Seyforth, a member of the health spa owned by Lee Causey.

In just two weeks, a phenomenal change took place in Mark's appearance and health. The usual side effects he had experienced while on other diets did not exist. Mark felt and looked wonderful. And he became so pleased with the diet, he wanted others to share his success.

My first involvement with the use of the protein milkshake as a meal-in-a-glass in a weight-reduction program was in 1976 when I became a consultant to Weight Loss International. Afterward I became a consultant and then research director for The Solgar Company in 1978.

My consulting for Weight Loss International gave me considerable experience with the problems of dieters. My research led me to develop an optimized program for fat loss which I published as *The Easy No-Flab Diet* (Marek, 1979). This was a nutritionally sound diet that concentrated on fat loss rather than weight loss or rapid loss.

However, it did not meet the needs of many people desiring a more rapid—but safe—weight loss combined with convenience and fat loss.

Joseph Perry, Research Director for Futuron Industries in Dallas, appreciated the special balance of complex carbohydrates, proteins, and fats in *The Easy No-Flab Diet* and suggested that the dinner meals from *The Easy No-Flab Diet* would be an improvement over the conventionally designed dinners used in conjunction with the milkshake diet.

Together, we have improved, if not perfected, the protein milkshake-plus-dinner diet. Modern motivational and behavioral modification techniques have also been incorporated, along with an outstanding exercise program. The combined program was given the name of The Slendernow Diet Program and introduced through the Slendernow Neighborhood Clubs of America. The experiences of these diet clubs and of all the previous protein-milkshake-plus-a-meal variations is the basis for this book.

This book endorses a total diet program rather than a particular segment or product. I am not now a consultant for the Slendernow Neighborhood Clubs of America or Futuron Industries, nor do I have any ties with them other than mutual respect and my appreciation for their help in making this diet program and book possible.

I hope this book helps you to achieve your goals in life and helps to bring you good health.

RICHARD PASSWATER
Ocean Pines, Maryland
February 1982

THE SLENDERNOW DIET

1

Lose weight with tasty, frothy, flavorful milkshakes and scrumptious meals. Is this another unhealthy fad diet? Seems too good to be true, but over 200,000 Americans from Hollywood to Bangor have shed unwanted pounds while improving their health with the remarkable Slendernow diet. This is not an experimental diet tried on a few individuals and then touted to the general public without adequate testing. The Slendernow Diet is the perfected evolution of the protein-enriched milkshake-dinner diet approach developed in 1975. We will discuss clinical trials, physician and nutritionist approvals, and other safety considerations later, but first, let's see if the Slendernow diet is for you.

There are probably thousands of variations of the basic four diets; low-calorie, fasts, modified fasts, and low-carbohydrate. You can lose weight with virtually any reducing diet provided you're not hungry (in which case you'll eventually eat more) and you find the menus varied and to your liking (otherwise, you won't stay on the diet long). No diet will succeed if it takes torturous willpower or bores you to death before you lose the desired weight.

A good diet should be nutritionally sound in terms of normal bodily needs, but also in regard to the special needs produced by the physical and emotional stresses of dieting itself.

A diet should provide a proper distribution of nutrients throughout the day to provide even nourishment and to prevent hunger pangs. Of course, calorie intake must be reduced below caloric expenditure so that stored fat is burned to meet the calorie deficit.

A good diet should not isolate the dieter from normal family or business activities and the foods should fit into regular meal patterns.

If you enjoy conventional and ethnic meals that include bread and butter, vegetables (including potatoes and buttered corn-on-the-cob), and various meats (vegetarian meals also included), then you'll actually enjoy the Slendernow Diet. Meals include spaghetti and meatballs with garlic bread, pizza, picnic basket fried chicken, and steak and potatoes. Feast on 34 delicious menus along with 101 rich, flavorful milkshake variations. Most recipes are provided. No exotic foods are required, nor extra preparation time. In fact, the milkshakes are faster and more convenient than most meals. No interruption of your lifestyle is required. You can have your business lunches or dinners, your parties and your dinner dates at restaurants. Also, you can picnic or stop at a fast-food restaurant.

You won't realize you're dieting unless you look in the mirror and see the results. The milkshakes and meals are so good you feel as if you are pampering yourself. There is no need for "rewards" for success in losing pounds and inches—you have taste treats every day.

And you can forget grapefruit, cottage cheese, carrots and celery unless you wish occasionally to add them to your meals.

Do you dislike counting calories or weighing food? No need to. The milkshake recipes and suggested food portions do that for you. Besides, the exact calorie count is not that critical—the point is, you'll be losing weight. And, since you won't be hungry, you have no temptation to cheat or overeat. In fact, hunger is so well satisfied, there is a temptation to skip a meal in the belief that it will help. Don't. The best results are achieved by eating your full daily quota.

Do you want more energy or a better complexion? The Slendernow Diet has done that for thousands of people. Many feel and look rejuvenated by the diet.

Do you need quick results to stay motivated? You will see results right from the start. However, after you have proven to yourself that you can lose weight very quickly on this diet, I will encourage you to moderate your rate of weight loss for the best long-term results. We don't want sagging skin or to see the pounds come back next year.

An overview of the Slendernow Diet program is that at breakfast you drink a meal-in-a-glass that contains the nutrients needed for energy and to prevent hunger until lunch. You simply add two tablespoons of a powdered balanced protein, one-half to one tablespoon of polyunsaturated oil, and flavoring to milk or your favorite juice.

This may not sound appetizing or filling to you but you're in for a very pleasant surprise. Indeed, it will fill you up without filling you out! The ingredients have been scientifically selected to complement each other in regard to the time they take to digest and nourish the body. Your blood sugar is always maintained at the proper level so that hunger is not triggered and you never have the "shakes," temper tantrums or depression common to diets that allow your blood sugar to become too low at times. On the other hand, the blend of carbohydrates, proteins, and fat is designed to prevent elevated blood sugar that would shut down the fat-burning process.

The Slendernow Diet does not produce the acid blood (ketosis) of very low carbohydrate diets. It is a moderate diet and should not be confused with extreme diets such as the liquid predigested protein diet. Sometimes people confuse the liquid predigested protein diet with protein milkshake diets. There is no similarity at all except that both diets have the word protein in their titles. The liquid predigested protein diet is a 400–600 calories diet consisting entirely of unbalanced, broken-down (fractionated) skin and hoof protein. The Slendernow Diet is a 1200–1500 calorie diet consisting of balanced, complete proteins, carbohydrates, and fats, including whole foods.

In the Slendernow Diet, we suggest you have your full 700–900 calorie meal at lunch. One of the problems contributing to fat production is that our society tends to eat a large dinner at the end of the day's activity. We should put the fuel into our body before we need the energy, not afterwards when it can only be converted to fat.

Those who enjoy business or social lunches will find it advantageous to have the regular meal at lunchtime. And if you live by yourself, eating a regular lunch out will mean no cooking or washing dishes at home.

Still, those who eat lunch alone may prefer to drink the second milkshake at lunchtime and have a full meal for dinner with the rest of the family or on a dinner date. This will not substantially alter the diet, and it is an acceptable alternative to the recommended program. Thus, you can arrange the two diet shakes (technically, protein-shakes or "pro-shakes" because they can be made without milk) and full meal to make you most comfortable.

You will find the alternating light and moderate exercises (walking and rebounding) shaping your figure as they speed your weight loss.

So then, if you're looking for a safe and proven diet that saves on your food bill, prevents hunger, boredom, tantrums, depression, nervousness, shakes, and a "drained" feeling and yet requires no exotic foods or extra preparation time or interruption of lifestyle—congratulations, you've found it!

One week on the Slendernow Diet and you will be pleased with yourself. But for optimizing your figure and developing the habits needed to maintain the figure you always wanted, please stay on the program for eight weeks. You've never dreamed it could be so easy.

You have already decided you want to shed your excess fat because of health or cosmetic reasons. If you decide that the Slendernow Diet is suited to your needs, please read on to learn more about the diet, rather than just turn to the menus. There is more to successful dieting than menus.

You should learn the importance of meal timing, meal size, proper eating habits, exercise, and how to avoid common dieting problems. If you understand the diet principles, you know what to expect and how to customize the diet to your individual needs and desires.

The next few chapters will discuss these important concepts in order to make the diet even easier.

You'll soon lose inches, your skin will glow, your hair and fingernails will take on a healthy luster, you'll feel a surge of vitality all day without a midday letdown. Thousands of satisfied dieters have claimed that this is undoubtedly the best reducing program ever developed.

2

Perhaps you're still not sure the Slendernow Diet is for you. After all, most people become interested in a diet plan only after they see dramatic results in their friends. Let me introduce you to a few friends kind enough to share their experiences with you. They too decided to try the Slendernow Diet (or an earlier variation) after witnessing the success of their friends. I hope their enthusiasm encourages you.

Their stories are chosen from several hundred sent to me because they illustrate how the Slendernow Diet* can help everyone—from the grossly overweight to the perfectionist wanting to shed those stubborn last five pounds. The best part of all is that they not only had success at weight loss, but as a bonus gained improved health and vitality, as well as a feeling that "life is better than ever." Looking good and feeling good do much for one's self-confidence and outlook on life.

I begin with a story that has a surprise ending. Mrs. Eron Shaw of Orlando, Florida, safely lost 40 pounds from her tiny-framed body and improved her health, but she has another very special reason for liking the Slendernow Diet. Well . . . let her tell the story.

> I'm very grateful to the friend who introduced me to the Slendernow Diet. In May 1978, I was carrying 145 pounds on my five-foot frame and size 4B feet.
>
> I was tired all the time and had frequent angina pains for which my doctor prescribed nitroglycerine. I felt achy and

*As mentioned in the preface, my experience with protein milkshakes goes back to 1957 and my association with reducing programs utilizing protein milkshakes-plus-a-dinner goes back to 1976. As the milkshake-dinner diets were improved, the name of the diet program was occasionally changed. For reading ease, I will refer to all properly designed milkshake-dinner diets with the generic description, the Slendernow Diet.

stiff, could not tie my shoes without feeling dizzy. It was so hard for me to bend over.

Less than four months later, I weighed 105 pounds and threw away my nitroglycerine pills. I went shopping for a new wardrobe and had a physical checkup. My doctor found absolutely nothing wrong with me. I feel great!

Most of all, I like the Slendernow Diet for saving my son's life or keeping him from being an invalid in a wheelchair for the rest of his life.

How did the Slendernow Diet save her son's life? Let Jim Shaw explain.

My first experience with the Slendernow Diet was in November of 1978. Having been a real hard-core fat person all my adult life and having gained and lost an incredible number of pounds over a 32-year span, my mother finally found something that really worked.

I had reached the prodigious weight of 490 pounds, had phlebitis in both legs which quickly turned into thrombosis with multiple blood clots in both legs.

I went to my doctor who immediately admitted me to a hospital where he prescribed bed rest and an anticoagulant. He advised me that if I did not lose a substantial amount of weight immediately, I would be dead in a matter of a few weeks, or at the very least, have both legs amputated. Quite frankly, I was scared to death.

After a ten-day stay in the hospital, I was released and I immediately started the Slendernow Diet. By the end of February 1979, I was down to 260 pounds. I can honestly say that the Slendernow Diet really works and is very effective for someone who simply wishes to maintain an even weight through the maintenance program.

Although protein milkshakes are very effective weight-loss aids, they cannot do it alone. For myself personally, it was a matter of reeducating my eating habits and realizing that my basal metabolism is extremely slow.

Jim sent along two pictures, one at 485 pounds and the other at 275 pounds. If Jim can do it, you can lose whatever you need to lose. It will certainly be easier for you. You have fewer pounds to lose and a faster basal metabolism. You'll feel so good about yourself after a few weeks on the Slendernow Diet that you'll be angry you waited this long to get started. Why miss any more fun because you have negative feelings about yourself because of your weight problem?

Was Jim's success a fluke? Not at all. I have many such success stories. Let me share another "gigantic" weight-loss success to make a point about how healthy the Slendernow Diet is.

Sharon D. (she doesn't want me to use her last name) of Atlanta also lost over 200 pounds on the Slendernow Diet. She explains.

> When I was a youngster, I contracted encephalitis. Following my illness, I started putting on weight. By the third grade, I weighed 133 pounds. Before the Slendernow Diet, my life was absolutely miserable.

At one point in Sharon's life, arthritis in her knees and hips became so severe that she walked with a cane. Her many pounds of excess weight kept her struggling and in constant pain. Sharon had difficulty in merely breathing. It was agony to simply walk from her office to the lunchroom. She had to have a special parking space reserved close to her office or she would have collapsed from exhaustion.

> Thanks to the Slendernow Diet, I no longer have arthritis pains. I go up and downstairs like nobody's business. Now I'm even called "speedy" at work. But one of my proudest days came when I told my boss I no longer needed that reserved parking place.

Sharon had tried other diets. While on one particular diet, Sharon claims it made her lose hair, teeth, her gall bladder and her equilibrium. She also remembers with horror the twenty-one days she spent in the hospital drinking only water.

Sharon concedes, "I did lose 30 pounds, but I lost almost as much just as fast on the Slendernow Diet and did it by eating the foods I love in the regular meals."

I trust these personal experiences illustrate that the Slendernow Diet is not only safe to stay on as long as you need to lose your excess weight, but it makes you healthier.

In case you are thinking that Jim and Sharon were young and resilient, and not subject to possible diet deficiencies, let me tell you about Kathleen Spalding who is 86 years old.

There was a time when Kathleen Spalding didn't worry about her weight. Fragile and feverish as a child, Kathleen's doctors always worried about her being excessively underweight. "Afer a long fever," explains Kathleen, "I was so thin and weak I could hardly move. My mother was told to feed me well and to keep me from overtiring. That meant no exercising—and a lot of extra food."

Although overpampering may have been necessary during her illnesses, it was this constant overpampering that also began Kathleen's dependence on food. Kathleen's fevers subsided as she grew older—but her eating pattern had already become well established. When a muscle disorder in Kathleen's eye dictated two major surgeries, and even more time off her feet, Kathleen sought comfort in food. Over the years, as she began to encounter other kinds of struggles, overeating continued to establish itself as a pattern. "I knew I was becoming overweight," admits Kathleen, "but I was always so active and busy that I thought my health was fine. Subconsciously, I guess it was possible I even thought all that food was what was keeping me healthy. It's certainly what my past had trained me to believe."

Although she was continually advised to lose weight, it wasn't until complications set in that Kathleen really began to take that advice seriously. "At one point, arthritis became so bad I was almost totally sapped of strength. My knees would hardly hold me up," remembers Kathleen. "I couldn't walk, hike, jog, or do any of the things I was used to doing. My antique shop suffered, and so did my sewing and painting. And my weight got up to 255 pounds!"

During her overweight years, Kathleen tried many diets; nearly every doctor she consulted prescribed a new one. "I can't say they didn't work," recalls Kathleen. "But they took such a painfully long time. It took me ten years to lose my first 75 pounds. And I was starving on an absolute minimum. After all those years of struggle, I still can't believe I lost my last 70 pounds on the Slendernow Diet in less than one year."

At this writing, at 4′ 10″ and 110 pounds, Kathleen Spalding is 86 years old—but claims to be 86 years young. An active member of many church and philanthropic clubs, Kathleen spends a lot of time in the community, or with friends. And she also gets plenty of exercise.

Low-Calorie Diets Didn't Work

If other diets were not successful for you, don't despair. Persons with sluggish metabolisms respond well to the Slendernow diet. I believe it is because of the improved nutrition that restores proper efficiency to your basal metabolism and hypothalamus.

Jim Shaw and Sharon D. both mentioned that very low-calorie diets did not help them. They felt like failures, but it wasn't their fault. Their very low-calorie diets were not nourishing them properly. They were not getting all the nutrients needed to build the enzymes that convert stored fat into available energy. Instead, their bodies had shifted gears into a slower metabolic rate to adjust to their reduced caloric intake.

Ordinarily women lose weight very nicely on 1200 calories a day, and men do just fine on 1500 calories a day. However, if the calories do not provide all of the required nutrients, weight loss is slowed or reversed.

Danice Boler of Shreveport, Louisiana, had just such a problem. Danice says her biggest accomplishment is being able to cross her legs again. Overweight for years, Danice lost 21 pounds in three weeks on the Slendernow Diet. Within five months, her weight loss measured 75 pounds and at final tally she had reduced from 209 pounds to 127 pounds.

> Before the Slendernow Diet, I had really come to believe the people who said they weren't eating and weren't losing weight," recalls Danice. "I've been to Weight Watchers and gained on 1500 calories a day. I've tried almost every kind of diet there is—once I even went on 800 calories a day for a year. I got depressed, my blood pressure dropped seriously, and my medical bills went sky high. I lost many of my reflexes—and total control of my left foot. I barely crawled

out of that year—it was the worst of my life. And through it all I only lost 24 pounds!

Danice was introduced to the Slendernow Diet at a friend's party. Although she was skeptical at first, her attitude soon changed. In six days Danice lost 12 pounds. It had taken her half a year to do that on 800 calories a day. Her Slendernow Diet was 1200 calories. Danice says,

> Now my weight is off for good. I've kept it off for a year and that's the way I intend to keep it. My doctor's bills are long paid and forgotten. I feel wonderful. The Slendernow Diet was like a miracle for me.

Mary Burkett of Pensacola, Florida, is another who found greater success with the Slendernow Diet than with very low-calorie diets.

> I had tried many diets, but I had never accomplished much. Once I had 600 calories a day for six weeks and lost only four pounds. I have lost 35 pounds and six inches from my waistline with the Slendernow Diet. My loss was steady and I experienced no hunger irritability.
>
> I lost inches all over—even in my arms and hands. I've lost three dress sizes. The Slendernow Diet has really changed my life.

Inches Melt Away

Mary Jo Norstorm was pleased.

> In 8 months I dropped 91 pounds of fat using the Slendernow Diet. I eliminated the high blood pressure medication which I had been using for years and yet my blood pressure reading is 110/70.

Carol Valen of Santa Barbara, California, writes,

> I've lost 90 pounds in 12 months, and gained energy and confidence. I feel great after fighting fat for 15 years.

Maurine Perone of Pleasant Hill, California, lost 62 pounds and 11 inches from her waistline. Maurine reports,

> Having been overweight all my life, I welcomed the opportunity to use a weight-loss program that had a sound nutritional basis. I lost 62 pounds in three and one-half months and never felt better.

In Temple Terrace, Florida, Mr. C. L. Brauhn lost 57 pounds and 6 inches from his waist.

> The Slendernow Diet did in six months what was impossible for years. In that time, I went from 215 to 158 pounds and 38″ to 32″ in the waist. I'm a new person thanks to the Slendernow Diet.

Of course, the waist isn't the only area to show weight loss. Here's the record kept by Albert Miller of Warren, Ohio. Notice that the weight was still off two years later.

	START	8 WEEKS	1 YEAR	2 YEARS
Weight	182	151	142	144
Waist	37.5	33	31.5	31
Hips	39.5	37.5	36	37
Thigh	23.5	21.5	20.5	20
Chest	39	35.5	34.5	34
Calf	14	13.25	13	12.5

Friends and relatives do notice the difference. Jeff S. of Concord, California, was convinced of the Slendernow Diet's effectiveness when he overheard his relatives raving about it.

> My aunt and uncle had just returned from a vacation in Fairbanks, Alaska. They were visiting their daughter who had lost 32 pounds on the Slendernow Diet in six weeks. They were so excited telling my parents about the program. I was in another room minding my own business, but I couldn't help but become interested.

At that time, I was 19 years old and weighed 265 pounds. I was so discouraged because I couldn't even buy the "in" styles in clothing like my friends. They only went to size 38 waist, and I wore a tight 44. My blood pressure was high and I knew I couldn't go on like this.

My mom and I decided to go on the program. I was pleased when I had my first shake. It was delicious tasting and it kept me from getting hungry for 4 to 5 hours. Now that is really something for me; really it was unbelievable! I was used to eating enormous meals and I had never been on a diet before.

I began to lose weight and inches. My friends began to notice my weight loss. My overweight friends would say, "Whatever it is, I want it!"

In five months on the Slendernow Diet, I have lost 52 pounds and am wearing size 38 pants. My blood pressure is down to normal.

Rapid Loss

Mark Combs of Jonesboro, Georgia, lost 40 pounds and eight inches from his waist. Charlie Browning of Ontario, Oregon, lost 35 pounds and six inches from his waist in 35 days. Charlie claims it's "the greatest thing that ever happened to me." Odell Miller of Gastonia, North Carolina, lost 35 pounds in 36 days. I wish they both had gone a little slower. Large men can safely lose at rapid rates, but small women should lose no faster than about 10 pounds in three weeks for the best results.

Holiday Feasts

Registered Nurse Mary Ellen Carlson of Minneapolis went from a size 10–12 to a 6–7 over the Thanksgiving to New Year's holiday period. While losing six inches from her waist, she went to many banquets and parties where she had meals like everyone else. Most people put on a few pounds over the festive holidays, but Slendernow Dieters can "enjoy" while losing weight.

Figure Shaping

Some diets take off pounds by temporarily increasing water loss from the body. People on such diets weigh less and are smaller in some areas, but essentially they look like smaller fat people rather than trim people. The Slendernow Diet pares away fat and firms the lean (muscle protein) tissue that shapes your figure.

Debbie Dempsey of Pensacola, Florida, explains,

> I lost 20 pounds in a month just by cutting down on food intake, but I only lost one dress size and my skin was sagging. I started the Slendernow Diet and have lost from size 15 to a size 7. My skin was very dry and now it's like baby skin. My hair was dry, now it's soft and shiny. I have more energy, I lost inches all over, and feel like I never have before.

Gail Borden of Clifton Park, New York, made steady progress from 153 to 125 pounds from May to October on the Slendernow Diet.

> The change in size is what really amazed me. I went from a size 16 to a 7–8. My daughter found that the balanced nutrition and exercise made her more alert. School became easier for her and she is in college full time and getting straight A's. Her new figure has recently attracted a new and exciting love in her life.

Energy and Well-Being

Everyone mentions in their letters that they have never felt better. Most mention that they have renewed energy.

Fred Crane of Safe, Missouri, writes,

> The Slendernow Diet's total nutrition program left me feeling like I did when I was 21. Previously, I had come home from work tired and run-down. Now I work my regular job, have a part-time sales job, run my photography business, and have an active social life. The Slendernow Diet has changed my whole outlook towards life.

Don Koester of Maitland, Florida, adds,

> I lost 20 pounds and 4 inches around my waist in one month on the Slendernow Diet. Best of all, my mental clarity was greatly sharpened, and I felt younger and more energetic than I had in years!

Elizabeth Hyde of Pleasant Hill, California, sums up the sense of pride that you can also experience.

> I love the Slendernow Diet program. It is the answer to my prayers. I have had a weight problem all my life. At 13 years of age, I weighed 170 pounds. I have lost 43 pounds in five months and have a freedom now I have never known. My two teenage girls are so proud of their mom—and so am I.

Elizabeth is proud of herself and you will be too after trying the Slendernow Diet. No diet is right for everyone in the world, but the Slendernow Diet has been right for many people in all walks of life—state governors, athletes, traveling salesmen, clergymen, housewives, and famous professional entertainers.

Now that you know that the Slendernow Diet program works, let's see what the doctors say about the diet.

3

Physicians not only approve of the Slendernow Diet, many physicians have chosen the diet for themselves and have recommended it highly for their patients. Physicians are very concerned about both being overweight and the methods used to reduce.

Obesity has been called our nation's number one malnutrition problem. We are becoming a nation of the overfed and undernourished. Many medical doctors believe that excessive weight can lead to many serious health disorders, including high blood pressure, diabetes, gall bladder and liver disease, osteoarthritis (from pressure of excess pounds on weight-bearing joints), and premature heart attack, which many believe to be the main killer of the obese. Definite proof of a cause-and-effect relationship has not been established between obesity and those diseases to satisfy everyone, but most physicians recognize obesity at least as a "risk factor" in the development of these diseases.

Physicians are very concerned about the harm to health that some fad diets can cause. The idea is to lose fat, not your health. Physicians would prefer that everyone lose weight the commonsense way just by cutting back a little at each meal on each of the food items. However, they have found that this works only for a few, much less than 5 percent. Hunger is not controlled and it is too tempting to eat an extra bite. Also, extra calories are disguised and consumed unknowingly.

Physicians realize that the average dieter wishes to go to bed fat and wake up thin and is therefore prey to crash diets. Crash diets stress the body chemistry, are usually nutritionally unbalanced, and, except in rare instances, produce only temporary results.

Physicians approve the Slendernow Diet because it provides weight reduction through controlled, well-balanced nutrition that reduces the number of calories consumed each day. Dr. John H. Ford, Jr., Professor, University of Miami School of Medicine, points out that "the protein powder has high biologic value and is blended with milk or juice. The milk or juice contains carbohydrate that prevents the loss of body-sugar stores so ketosis and acidosis do not occur. Further carbohydrate is supplied by the regular dinner eaten each day. Fat is supplied by the dinner and the polyunsaturated oil added to the protein milkshakes. There is no doubt that a small amount of fat is necessary in the diet to provide the essential fatty acids the body cannot produce and to aid in the absorption of the essential fat-soluble vitamins A, D, E, and K. Vitamin and mineral supplements help prevent vitamin deficiency and possible electrolyte imbalance due to reduced food intake."

It is the total nutritional balance of the Slendernow Diet that provides it with a wide margin of safety. The moderate calorie (1200 for women, 1500 for men) intake produces the optimal rate of weight loss. The Slendernow Diet is moderate and well balanced and proven to be safe and effective. This is why physicians recommend it.

Before discussing the results of controlled clinical trials, let's look at what several doctors have to say about the diet. (Because physicians frown on publicity, I will use only their initials.)

Medical doctors sometimes have weight problems too. Long hours, little exercise, frustrations and all of the problems that cause creeping weight gain affect everyone. Several physicians have lost considerable weight on the Slendernow Diet, and also recommend it to their patients.

Dr. W. B., an anesthesiologist in Winchester, Ohio, writes,

> I endorse the Slendernow Diet wholeheartedly. I have lost 135 pounds on the Slendernow Diet! My wife has lost 65 pounds! I recommend Slendernow to my patients, not just because it is so well balanced, but because it is so uncomplicated and easy to use. People can even go off it for a day or two without losing any of its positive results.

Dr. T. L. of Yuba City, California, tried the Slendernow Diet while he was serving as medical director for the County Hospital.

> I lost 60 pounds on the Slendernow Diet. What really strengthens my endorsement of the Slendernow Diet is the health benefits. After I'd been on the program a few weeks, my blood pressure dropped to normal. Many of my patients who'd been suffering from diabetes, hypoglycemia, high blood pressure and elevated blood fats were able to reduce or discard medical prescriptions.
>
> The Slendernow Diet is simple and fast. It's so satisfying that it lends that extra support needed in early dieting stages.

Dr. R. B. is an obstetrician and gynecologist in Elk Grove Village, Illinois, and writes,

> I believe the Slendernow Diet provides for better nutritional weight control than the overwhelming majority of Americans have previously experienced. And I also believe that simultaneously, it leads to better health.
>
> I chose the Slendernow Diet, among many alternatives, after undergoing open heart surgery. In four months, I lost 52 pounds. I would go out of my way to recommend this program for any patients with existing heart conditions.

Dr. J. V. is a cardiovascular surgeon in Roseville, California. He hasn't had a weight problem himself, but knows all about the problems of dieting.

> I am very enthusiastic about the quality of the Slendernow Diet. I deal with many overweight patients, and obesity is one of the main risk factors in their cardiovascular problems. I recommend the Slendernow Diet to help them lose weight and save money—I tell them that if they don't lose weight, I'll charge them by the pound for my services!
>
> Those who follow the program lose weight safely and effectively. One patient lost 12 pounds the first week and another lost 35 pounds in seven weeks. My wife and my brother-in-law also have lost quite a lot of weight on the program.

Dr. J. V. has recommended the Slendernow Diet to other physicians. One of his colleagues, Dr. R. C., who specializes in internal medicine and gastroenterology in Roseville, states,

One of my colleagues introduced me to the Slendernow Diet. I find it a very effective weight reduction program.

I have several hundred patients on the program. They lose weight safely. Some of these patients are special cases and the balanced nutrition of the Slendernow Diet has been outstanding in relieving their conditions. One diabetic patient, for example, lost weight on the Slendernow Diet and now totally controls the diabetes with a single pill and no insulin. Another patient had such a high blood-sugar level that I considered hospitalization for treatment until the Slendernow Diet stabilized her metabolism and lowered the level of sugar in her blood.

Before the Slendernow Diet, I ignored treating obesity. It was such a difficult problem to deal with. On other programs, weight often is lost with such difficulty and found again with such ease, that I'm troubled when I see persons losing five pounds and gaining back ten. The Slendernow Diet maintenance program is easy. And it works. One or two shakes a week in place of empty high-calorie foods, for example, helps insure both sound nutrition and that ideal weight.

I don't need to diet, but I enjoy the taste of the shakes and the knowledge that they provide food for more than just thought. I share the successes and joys of weight reduction with my patients who use the Slendernow Diet, and that pleases me most.

Dr. C. M. of Fort Worth adds,

The Slendernow Diet is doing something now about the current menace of obesity. I lost 19 pounds using the Slendernow Diet and use the milkshakes off and on for maintenance.

The Slendernow Diet is the most complete of the natural weight-control programs. It lets people enjoy the benefits of sound nutrition at the same time they're taking off unwanted, unhealthy pounds and inches.

Those on the Slendernow Diet upon my recommendation feel confident about the program because they know it's good for them. They feel great on the program, too, and for good reason. I am firmly convinced that the excellent nutrition of the Slendernow Diet program makes you brighter and more alert, and helps reduce the nervous tension that normally accompanies dieting. I believe that the Slendernow Diet program used as directed could significantly reduce the incidence of heart disease.

I like the versatility of the Slendernow Diet. It satisfies the physical and psychological needs associated with weight reduction. The main meal is an integral part of the program. It provides the bulk to balance out the other nutrients and the variety to spice up the diet. Different flavorings added to the milkshakes or juice-shakes can also lend variety.

I like the built-in advantage of the Slendernow Diet that helps to modify poor eating habits. The milkshakes are easy to prepare, taste great and are easy to stay on. Anyone wanting to maintain his weight can simply decrease the use of the milkshakes and increase the consumption of well-balanced regular meals.

You lose weight and feel great on the Slendernow Diet—that's the bottom line.

Dr. M. M., an obstetrician and gynecologist in Columbus, Ohio, reveals,

I realized the Slendernow Diet to be extremely good when I lost 30 pounds on it myself. The Slendernow Diet is easy to follow; it's a program that gets results.

I feel that the Slendernow Diet is basically a complete program. The basic requirements, in fact, are more than adequately met. *The Slendernow Diet is probably the greatest weight reduction regimen formulated for general use in terms of overall quality nutrition.*

I recommend the Slendernow Diet to my patients. The ease of the program, furthermore, produces motivation, and motivation yields results. Once their weight stabilizes, I encourage my patients to continue with at least one milkshake a day.

I personally drink two shakes daily and then eat a well-balanced evening meal. This program satisfies my eating needs. The entire program is so fulfilling that it keeps you from going back to bad habits. We all "cheat" once in a while. The Slendernow Diet is probably the only regimen on which you can cheat a bit and still not endanger your program.

How about its use for children? Dr. H. B. is a pediatrician in Hendersonville, Tennessee. She comments,

The Slendernow Diet works. It's been proven. I have personally lost weight on the Slendernow Diet. And I feel great! I recommend the Slendernow Diet to many of my patients over 13 years of age. My husband also shares my enthusiasm. As a dentist, he's convinced the Slendernow Diet can help his patients.

And speaking of dentists, Richard H. Bond, D.M.D., of Conway, South Carolina, has an interesting story to tell.

When I started the Slendernow Diet three years ago, I weighed 310 pounds. I lost 120 pounds in the first year. My current weight is 187 pounds.

Before the Slendernow Diet, I tried numerous other programs, including things such as diet pills (Preludin during my teen years). Pills worked for a while—but once I went off them, I always regained the weight. So-called diet shots and diet sheets had the same effects. It wasn't until the Slendernow Diet that I saw results—and I am continuing to see results.

When I began the Slendernow Diet, I found that I had more energy than I had before. I still feel terrific—and I haven't regained any weight. The Slendernow Diet has changed my life in many many ways.

One of the most amusing things to have happened to me since losing weight is not being recognized by people who know me. I have been asked if I am Dr. Bond's son, for instance. Patients have asked—after I have examined them—if they could have Dr. Bond check them instead of his new associate. And one local merchant and fellow Kiwanis Club member (who prides himself on knowing everyone) conversed with me for several minutes before finally asking who I was. His embarrassment was very apparent.

I endorse the Slendernow Diet wholeheartedly—and I hope that many others will know the triumph that it has given to me.

Clinical Test

A producer of one of the protein powders used for the protein milkshake and juice-shakes had the two-shakes-a-day-plus-dinner diet plan tested as an in-patient study at the metabolic research unit of a major teaching hospital. The clinical trial confirmed moderate but consistent weight loss averaging 11 pounds over a three-week period. All relevant clinical and laboratory parameters were monitored, including blood and urine tests. The blood tests included a glucose, BUN, creatinine, sodium, potassium, chloride, carbon dioxide, uric acid, calcium, phosphorus, protein, albumin, AKP, SGOT, WBC, RBC, hemoglobin and hematocrit. The urine tests included glucose, acetone, protein and pH.

No untoward effects were observed. The diet was well accepted by the subjects and patient compliance was excellent.

That's what doctors think about the Slendernow Diet and what the clinical trial confirmed. Now here's what a few dieters discovered about their health while on the Slendernow Diet.

Blood Pressure

Lois E. of Eugene, Oregon, reports,

I'd tried some of the fad diets with no lasting results. I went on the Slendernow Diet. When I lost ten pounds, my husband announced that he would go on the milkshakes too.

Because he was under the doctor's care for high blood pressure, my answer was, "No, you need your doctor's OK." Unknown to me, he had already asked his doctor. The doctor was on the Slendernow Diet himself!

After my husband started on the Slendernow Dict, his blood pressure came down fast. After being on the strongest form of medication that he could take, he is now on a very mild form. He maintains normal readings.

I tell people that the Slendernow Diet has changed our lives, but really it has saved our lives.

Junius F. of Richmond, Virginia, lost 45 pounds in 60 days.

I lost 9 inches in the waist, 4 inches in the chest, 7 inches in the hips and a full 2 inches in the neck. I also was successful in bringing my blood pressure down from 195/120 to 120/60 during this time. Before going on the Slendernow Diet, I had considerable back pain and associated problems. I no longer have any back problems. In fact, my total health has improved considerably.

Cholesterol

Fred Mouzon of Huntsville, Alabama, weighed 198 pounds and had a 39-inch waist. His cholesterol level was 360 (normal range is *150–280*). In two-and-a-half months, he lost 25 pounds and 6 inches from his waist. His cholesterol level dropped over 100 points during that time. His wife Ruth also lost 12 pounds during that time.

Earlier in this chapter, I reported that doctors use the Slendernow Diet to lower cholesterol and high blood pressure.

Injuries and Overweight Complications

Injuries can cause people to become less active and thus overweight. As a result, their health can deteriorate and their pain increase. Such unfortunate individuals have to be especially on guard against unbalanced fad diets that could weaken them further. Many dieters have written to say that they went on the Slendernow Diet because it was so balanced nutritionally and easy to follow. As a result, they broke the vicious cycle that was aggravating their conditions and were able to overcome their original problem as well as their overweight problem. To these persons, there is no doubt that the Slendernow Diet is a very, very healthful diet. Here's a typical case as an illustration. Rich Bell tells his story.

I began the Slendernow Diet when I weighed 252 pounds, was bedridden and an invalid due to a back injury. I was depressed, tired, apathetic, and hungry all the time. Within seven weeks, my weight was down to 175 pounds.* No longer was I bedridden or depressed. Vitality and health were surging through me. Slendernow created for me a new way of living. One based upon nutritional feelings balanced by moderate exercise due to my excess energy created from the Slendernow Diet Program. Slendernow saved my life. I recommend it heartily to one and all.

It's difficult to imagine the problems brought about by injuries complicated by weight gain.

Imagine arthritis so severe it forces someone to retire on disability. Imagine barely being able to walk, sleeping only two or three hours a night, living on countless pain killers. To make this nightmare almost unbearable, she is thirty to forty pounds overweight—but doesn't have the strength to do anything about it.

Imagine her husband being caught beneath the undercarriage of a train—crippled almost beyond recovery. Having been critically injured, the doctors gave him only two years to live, unless he ceased all activity. He is forced to retire on disability and to complicate his problems almost beyond endurance—he is dangerously overweight. He is backed into a corner. Unable to exercise. Unable to afford the nutritionally balanced meals he requires.

Perhaps you can imagine these things, perhaps not. But Bill and Lydia Strawn of Norfolk, Virginia, had to live them first-hand. Lydia was forced to retire from her job because of severe arthritis. Bill had his accident in 1967. Both were so ill—and so overweight—that they felt nothing could help them to regain their health. But then the Strawns claim to have been introduced to a lifestyle that would affect their physical and mental well-being—helping to transform them into healthy, active, and alert human beings.

It was a visit to Florida that brought this incredible change. At Christmas of 1975, the Strawns drove to Florida to visit their son.

* The Slendernow Diet can be used for this rapid a weight loss by eating smaller meals than recommended. However, such rapid weight loss is not advisable.

> When he opened the car door, recalls Lydia, I nearly passed out at the weight he had lost. My son had lost 60 pounds on the Slendernow Diet. His weight had dropped from 310 pounds to 250 pounds. I decided to start the Slendernow Diet the very next day.
>
> Within one week after starting the diet, I had come off all my pain pills and I haven't taken one since. Within a month I was walking just like in the old days before my arthritis and by two months I had lost 37 pounds.

It didn't take long for Bill to take notice of his wife's progress. Adopting the Slendernow Diet program himself, he lost 39 pounds in two months. Bill claims to have remained in excellent health ever since.

Pregnancy

The true mark of the soundness of a diet is whether a physician will prescribe it during pregnancy. The nutritional needs during pregnancy are considerably greater than otherwise. *Never* go on a diet without your doctor's approval if there is any chance that you are pregnant!

I do not recommend any diet to anyone during pregnancy. That is a matter for your physician. However, as noted earlier in this chapter, several obstetricians and gynecologists have recommended the Slendernow Diet to their patients. In some cases, the Slendernow Diet has been recommended during pregnancy.

Alicia Baugher of Jax, Florida, writes,

> I followed the Slendernow Diet program for nine months while pregnant with the approval of my gynecologist. I gained a total of seventeen pounds during this pregnancy. During my first pregnancy, I gained 44 pounds, and during my second pregnancy, I gained 38 pounds.
>
> Also, during this pregnancy, I had no morning sickness or vomiting as with the other two. We had a natural childbirth in the hospital on Saturday and out on Monday morning. I had a very healthy 8-pound 5-ounce baby boy. I am currently breast-feeding my baby and still taking the milkshakes twice a day in lieu of two meals. Doctors say our baby is a

> picture of health. After two months he has gained seven pounds and grew 4½ inches.

Keep in mind the milkshakes are nutritious and can always be used as a healthy diet supplement as Jerilyn Benson of North Myrtle Beach, South Carolina, writes.

> I am a vegetarian and my obstetrician was afraid I would not get enough protein in my diet when I was pregnant. I drank Slendernow Diet milkshakes through two pregnancies and two years of breast feeding. Both my babies were extremely healthy and alert, and I had beautiful natural deliveries, with no complications. My doctor was very pleased with the results.
>
> Incidentally, I never developed an overweight condition.

What better testimony to the safety of the Slendernow Diet could there be? Physicians and their patients have documented their approval for your benefit. Now let's look at the sound nutrition behind the effective Slendernow Diet.

4

Nutritionists are very skeptical about diets. They have seen many that can be dangerous. Although no one really knows how much harm some fad diets have done, it seems as if two or three potentially harmful fad diets are introduced each year.

Nutritionists are very much involved with proper nourishment and eating habits. Some cannot understand why people simply can't control their weight by cutting back a little at each meal. These nutritionists forget that the rest of the world is not that involved in nutrition and as a result learn bad habits that are hard to break. It is human nature to want to go on a crash diet, lose weight, and then go back to the same bad habits that put on those extra pounds in the first place.

The Slendernow Diet is sound nutritionally and it does reeducate the dieter in terms of proper meal sizes and combinations. The success in keeping the weight off is largely due to following the complete eight-week program, even if the desired weight loss is achieved earlier than that.

However, if you run up to a typical nutritionist and announce that you are on a powdered-protein milkshake diet—look out; he'll boil over! Another Fad Diet! You don't *need* that much protein!

The Slendernow Diet is a very sensible, safe, and effective program. What you *need* is to lose your extra weight safely. You also need a program that is pleasant and convenient.

What the nutritionist needs is to forget his prejudice against anything else except cutting back at each meal (and being hungry all day), and to look at the details of the diet.

When the details are examined, nutritionists are amazed. As nutritionist Carol Koester of Orlando, Florida, writes,

I had been teaching nutrition classes for 20 years when I first heard the unbelievable claims about the Slendernow Diet. Wanting to expose another fad, and perhaps protect some of the unwary public, I analyzed the complete program. I was amazed! Here was what appeared to be perfectly balanced nutrition.

Still with some reservations, I tried it myself. I lost 15 pounds and two dress sizes in three weeks. My muscle tone improved, and my energy level soared. After getting down to my desired weight, I have continued to drink delicious Slendernow Diet shake for breakfast nearly every day of my life. It helps round out my nutrition for the entire day, and helps me stay in shape.

Even if you are not a nutritionist, you should *know* that the Slendernow Diet will improve your health. This chapter provides the details of the excellent nourishment provided by the Slendernow Diet for your examination.

Needed Calories

When you reduce your calorie intake below that of your calorie expenditure, you will lose weight; your body supplies the missing calories by "burning" its own tissue. Most people assume that all of the missing calories are provided by burning body fat. This is not necessarily so.

Your body can convert only a given amount of fat into energy in a day. There are several steps involved in mobilizing body fat and converting it to energy. Each step in the process is controlled by a specific enzyme. Since the body has been adding to its fat reserves, fat-producing enzymes are abundant, but fat-burning enzymes are scarce. The body doesn't waste energy and materials by building enzymes it doesn't use.

You can't force your body to burn more fat than it's capable of burning, no matter how little you eat or how great the calorie deficit is. Once your calorie intake has been reduced to the limit for the effective conversion of body fat to energy, any further calorie reduction will only cause your lean (muscle and organ) tissue to be burned. A fast can result in burning more lean tissue than fat tissue. Two-thirds of the weight lost on starvation diets is lean tissue. Oh, yes, you lose weight—but when you begin eating agan, the body strives to rebuild its debilitated lean tissue, and the weight returns even though you are not overeating.

The Slendernow Diet provides adequate calories and protein to maintain the lean tissue, while causing stored body fat to be consumed. Most nutritionists agree that 1200 calories a day for women, and 1500 calories a day for men are optimal for weight-loss programs. The rate of loss provided by this calorie intake depends on how overweight the person is to begin with.

Protein, Protein, Why Protein

Why add protein powder to the diet shakes? Why not add powdered complex carbohydrates or a mixture of complex carbohydrates and protein?

Complex carbohydrate serves mainly as fiber or bulk to keep things moving along our digestive tract. Dietary fiber is important, but it is not as important as protein. In fact, balanced protein powder usually contain both protein and carbohydrate. A blend that I prefer is about 80 percent protein, 10 percent digestible carbohydrate, and the remainder mineral and nondigestible fiber.

Complex carbohydrate and high-fiber diets are currently very popular, but it is difficult in using them to design a varied, nutritionally sound diet that is also appetizing and convenient. Few apparently "healthy" overweight persons decide to remain on such diets sufficiently long enough to lose their extra pounds; those sufficiently motivated by fear of death from heart disease or those who prefer semi-vegetarian low-fat diets can tolerate such diets very well. These persons, however, are not the typical dieters.

A high-complex-carbohydrate diet really works only when whole foods are eaten. Convenient nutritious milkshakes cannot be made from powdered bran or sawdust. Now let's look at the reasons for insuring that the protein needs are met.

Next to water, protein is the most abundant substance in the body. It's the building material for all the cells and enzymes.

Not all protein is the same. The usefulness or quality of a protein depends on its balance of subunits (building blocks) called amino acids. Our bodies contain 22 different amino acids, made out of eight basic amino acids. We must obtain these basic eight amino acids in our diet; thus they are called *essential* amino acids.

Protein quality is measured by how well the protein is incorporated into the body. One useful measurement of protein quality is the Protein Efficiency Ratio (PER). Milk protein contains an excellent balance of all the essential amino acids and is called a "complete" protein. Milk protein (casein), with a PER of 2.5, is the standard by which other proteins are compared. Egg protein is higher (3.5 +) and soybean protein is lower (2.0). However, when proteins are mixed, they may complement each other in amino acid content and thus boost their PER. The optimal PER rating for a protein powder supplement is 2.5 to 3.0.

Powdered protein is a carefully controlled protein source, created from soybean and milk sources, designed specifically to provide you with protein. Like animal protein, it provides all of the essential and necessary ingredients to supply the body's needs. Unlike natural animal protein, however, it does not provide hidden fat to the body. Meat contains fat in each cell, not just the fat you can see around the edges.

Liquid predigested protein has a negative PER (– 1.2) and is an incomplete protein that cannot support growth at low calorie levels. No wonder it caused great concern when it was used as the exclusive ingredient of a reducing diet.

It is important to realize that protein is needed daily for body repair and body function. The body can convert excess protein into carbohydrates and fats, but protein cannot be made from carbohydrate or fat. Protein cannot be stored in the body. Protein can only be made from protein.

The amount of protein recommended daily has been established by the Food and Nutrition Board of the National Academy of Sciences as 65 grams for the adult male and 55 grams for the adult female.

My point is that "need" implies the amount required for a healthy existence. The Slendernow Diet provides more than the minimum amount required for average health, but it does not supply too much of anything. The average American diet provides too much—too much fat and too many calories. The Slendernow Diet reduces the fat and carbohydrate levels in order to reduce calories. It maintains the protein needed to maintain your lean tissue in best health.

If your diet slips to near the minimal protein levels, your thought processes can be hindered. Amino acids such as tryptophan and phenylalanine are essential ingredients of the neurotransmitters (chemicals that carry nerve impulses between nerve cells). The amino acid glutamine can be converted in brain cells to glutamic acid and then into energy for the brain. Your mental and emotional well-being depends on meeting your highest need of protein—not your lowest need for existence.

Without sufficient protein, your skin will wrinkle and sag, and your hair and nails will suffer as well. You may remain alive on lower protein levels, but you may be healthier on more protein than 55 or 65 grams per day. However, once you do satisfy your protein needs for optimal health, extra protein is of no special value and will be converted to carbohydrate or fat by the body. The protein in the Slendernow Diet is not converted to fat, because any extra protein could be burned for energy due to the calorie deficit.

There is nothing magic about protein powder except that it assures meeting all of your dietary needs for the largest single substance in your body and is convenient to use and pleasant tasting. The Slendernow Diet works because the calorie content of the diet is lowered, while nutrition is improved. Protein is not dangerous, or we couldn't eat high-protein foods such as fish, poultry, meat, milk, eggs, or soybeans.

Diet Shake Nutrition

The critical component of the Diet Shakes is the protein powder, but it is not the only component. Tables 4.1 and 4.2 summarize the major nutrients and calories of the two daily Diet Shakes, but keep in mind that the shakes also provide vitamins and minerals.

TABLE 4.1

Major Nutrients in Two Diet Milkshakes

	CALORIES	PROTEIN (GRAMS)	CARBOHYDRATE (GRAMS)	FAT (GRAMS)
4 tablespoons protein powder	140	30	5	trace
1 tablespoon oil	126	0	0	14
16 oz. skim milk	180	18	24	0
2 Milkshake Total	446	48	29	14

TABLE 4.2

Major Nutrients in one Diet Juice-Shake and one Diet Milkshake

	CALORIES	PROTEIN (GRAMS)	CARBOHYDRATE (GRAMS)	FAT (GRAMS)
4 tablespoons protein powder	140	30	5	trace
1 tablespoon oil	126	0	0	14
8 oz. orange juice	110	2	26	0
8 oz. skim milk	90	9	12	0
One Juice-shake & One Skim Milkshake Total	466	41	43	14

Main Meal Nutrition

The main meal, whether it is eaten at lunch or dinner, should average 750 calories for women and 1050 calories for men. The meals typically contribute 40–70 grams of protein, 55–90 grams of carbohydrate, and 15–30 grams of fat. Complex carbohydrates are stressed in the main meals.

The main meals have also been analyzed for their potassium, sodium, magnesium, calcium and phosphorus content. Table 4.3 lists typical meal mineral content. In addition, a multiple vitamin and mineral supplement is required. Thus, a balanced nutritional program is supplied.

TABLE 4.3

Mineral Content of the Main Meal

MINERAL	MILLIGRAMS
Potassium	1900–2500
Sodium	300–1000
Magnesium	150–210
Calcium	570–650
Phosphorus	650–1000

TABLE 4.4

Two Diet Milkshakes plus typical Main Meals

	CALORIES	PROTEIN (GRAMS)	CARBOHYDRATE (GRAMS)	FAT (GRAMS)
Two Diet Milkshakes	446	48	29	14
Typical Main Meal	750	57	80	23
Total	1196	105	109	37

TABLE 4.5

Diet Juice-shake plus Diet Milkshakes plus Main Meal

	CALORIES	PROTEIN (GRAMS)	CARBOHYDRATE (GRAMS)	FAT (GRAMS)
Juice- and Milkshakes	466	41	43	14
Typical Main Meal	750	57	80	23
Total	1216	98	123	37

TABLE 4.6

Typical American Diet

YEAR	CALORIES	PROTEIN (GRAMS)	CARBOHYDRATE (GRAMS)	FAT (GRAMS)
1910	3480	102	492	125
1950	3230	95	403	140
1976	3300	101	376	157

Source: Page, L. and Friend, B., *BioScience* 28(3) 194 (1978).

Total Nutrition

Tables 4.4 and 4.5 show the values for the major nutrients for the combined Diet Shakes and main meal. Compare these values to those in Table 4.6 which is what the so-called "average" person is eating. You will note that the protein content of each is the same, but calories are reduced in the Slendernow Diet as carbohydrates are cut from 376 to 110–120 grams, and fat is reduced from 157 grams to 37 grams.

Your total intake of vitamins and minerals will depend on the amount used to fortify the protein powder and the amount in the multiple vitamin and mineral supplement. It is not unreasonable to expect the protein powder to be fortified so that when combined with milk, two servings provide the recommended dietary allowances of each vitamin and mineral.

5

Now that you've decided the Slendernow Diet is for you, let's make sure your health status is compatible with the Slendernow Diet. Don't even think of dieting—on any diet—without checking with your physician. Of course, the Slendernow Diet is safe, but dieting itself may be bad for *your* physical or emotional health.

All you have to do is call your doctor. He knows *you* well enough to advise you over the phone, but he may want to check you and ask you to come in for an examination. He realizes that you will be in better health at your ideal weight, but if you have a liver or kidney problem, this may not be the best time to correct the weight problem. Are you able to exercise moderately? Are you allergic to any of the foods?

The Slendernow Diet is compatible with patients having heart disease, diabetes, hypoglycemia, high blood pressure, arthritis and most other diseases. If you have gout, the 100 grams of protein in the Slendernow may or may not be too much for you and may contribute to uric acid buildup. Your physician may wish to monitor your uric acid level as you proceed with the diet.

Emotional health is important too. Is your life fairly serene? Trying to do too much at once or trying to change too much at once may cause emotional problems.

If you have no health problems which preclude you from dieting, your physician will want to know what diet you plan to use. Explain to him that the Slendernow Diet is highly recommended by physicians and is a moderate, balanced-nutrition program. Important information for your doctor is that the diet has 1200 calories per day for women and 1500 calories a day for men. It is a reduced fat and carbohydrate diet, providing 100 grams of protein, 115 grams of carbohydrate, and 37 grams of fat per day on the 1200-calorie diet.

It is accomplished by substituting high-protein, balanced amino acid milkshakes for two meals a day while eating a balanced main meal of 750 to 1050 calories for the third. Tell your physician you will also be taking a multiple vitamin and mineral pill as insurance.

That's it. A quick call to your physician and you're all set. What if you don't check? It's gambling! You want to lose weight, not your health. Don't play the odds. You are unique, a wonderful individual person. Don't become a statistic because you didn't check with a doctor first.

6

You will have the greatest success in dieting if you set a goal. Yes, you can lose weight without setting a goal, but the temptation to stop before you reach perfection is too great. However, you should set a reasonable goal. The problem is to determine just what is a reasonable goal for you.

Weight charts can be confusing and misleading. Rely less on them than on the mirror. The mirror can't tell you exactly how many pounds you need to lose, but the mirror does tell you when you should diet and when you reach perfection.

A better indicator of the amount of body fat you need to lose is the pinch test. But the pinch test doesn't tell you how many pounds you need to lose either. The pinch test tells you when you need to lose weight and when you reach perfection. One advantage of the pinch test over the mirror is that you can measure your progress more easily.

The same can be said of the measuring tape. It's great for measuring your progress, and you know when you reach your goal when your old clothes fit again. But the tape, too, doesn't tell you how many pounds you need to lose.

How then do you set your goal? How about trying to reach the weight you were at age 25—provided you were trim then.

Yes, set your ultimate goal at your "age 25" weight. Also set a goal to be able to fit into the same clothes size you were then.

You should also set subgoals at five-pound intervals. Every time you reach a subgoal, reward yourself, not with extra food, but with a present. Subgoals and reward strategy will be discussed later.

Now that you have set your goal, you should set a reasonable time allowance as to when you should reach this goal. If you determine that you need to lose 20 pounds, don't try to do it in a week. Remember, if you lose weight too fast, you will lose vital lean tissue and your figure, strength and health will suffer. In addition, when you switch to a maintenance diet, your body will rebuild the lean tissue and much of the lost weight will return.

A reasonable goal of weight loss is to lose 3–7 pounds the first week, 2–5 pounds the second week, and 1½ to 3 pounds every week thereafter. Thus in three weeks a large, moderately overweight person should lose 15 pounds, and a small, barely overweight person should lose 6½ pounds. The weight loss in the clinical trial mentioned in Chapter 3, involving all types of people, averaged 11 pounds per person in three weeks. The person with more than 50 pounds to lose can easily lose more than 20 pounds safely. True, some of the examples given in Chapter 2 told of dieters losing at a faster rate, but as I have mentioned, I prefer people to lose more slowly. It's easier on them and longer lasting.

Be kind to yourself when you set your goal. Allow for an occasional plateau or temporary fluctuation. If you are on the small side and less than 20 pounds overweight, set your goal by dividing the number of pounds you want to lose by 2. This is the *maximum* number of weeks to allow yourself to reach your goal. During this period you will be on target if you lose between 1½ to 3 pounds each week after the first two weeks. If you lose at an appreciably faster rate after the first two weeks, add more food to your main meal. If your weight loss is slower, cut some calories from your main meal.

If you are larger and have more than 20 pounds to lose, set your time limit by dividing the number of pounds you want to lose by 3. This is the maximum number of weeks to allow yourself to reach your goal. During this period, you will be on target if you lose between 2 to 5 pounds every week after the first two weeks. Again, if weight loss is appreciably faster than this, add more food to your main meal, and if slower, cut a few calories from the main meal.

Remember, weight loss differs from person to person, but the typical dieter will lose weight faster at the beginning of a diet. Some of this initial weight loss can represent water loss and reduced bulk in the intestinal tract. This seems to happen more frequently in those who cut back on food in the main meal. If they start burning lean tissue because the calorie deficit is greater than can be made up by burning mobilized body fat, water loss is appreciable. Of course, the greatly reduced food intake further reduces the bulk in the diet.

As you approach your goal, the rate of weight loss will start to slow. When this happens, you can reduce the food in the main meal by 150–200 calories to speed up the process, or you can continue on to your goal at the slower rate. You will reach your goal in any event.

Use Table 6.1 to plot your weight progress toward your goal.

When you reach a stubborn plateau, where weight seems to stay the same for several days, you can jolt your metabolism by going on three milkshakes, with no main meals, for a day, and repeating this again two days later if necessary.

Plateaus are usually caused when water is being retained in the cells in place of the fat that was removed, or when the body is retaining water due to increased salt intake or monthly menstrual cycle changes. Sometimes the plateaus mark the period when the amount of muscle tissue being built through the exercise program equals the amount of weight being lost from the fat cells. The net result is no change in weight, but a change in the waistline and other areas.

Sometimes the plateau is not really a plateau, but an apparent plateau caused by inaccurate weighings. One week you record a weight lower than it really is, and the next week you record a weight slightly higher than it really is.

Standardize your weighing procedure as much as possible. Weigh yourself before breakfast. Make three separate weighings and take the average. Get off the scale and on again each time. Watch the scale to make sure it returns precisely to zero when you get off. If it doesn't, reset, and repeat the procedure.

Your progress can also be noted by the increase in firmness of certain areas as the flabbiness disappears.

The best way to monitor your progress is to keep a weekly record of weight loss, inches lost, and flabbiness. Tables 6.1, 6.2, and 6.3 are for your use in following your progress.

TABLE 6.1

Weight-Loss Progress Toward Goal

Starting Weight ______ Target Weight ______

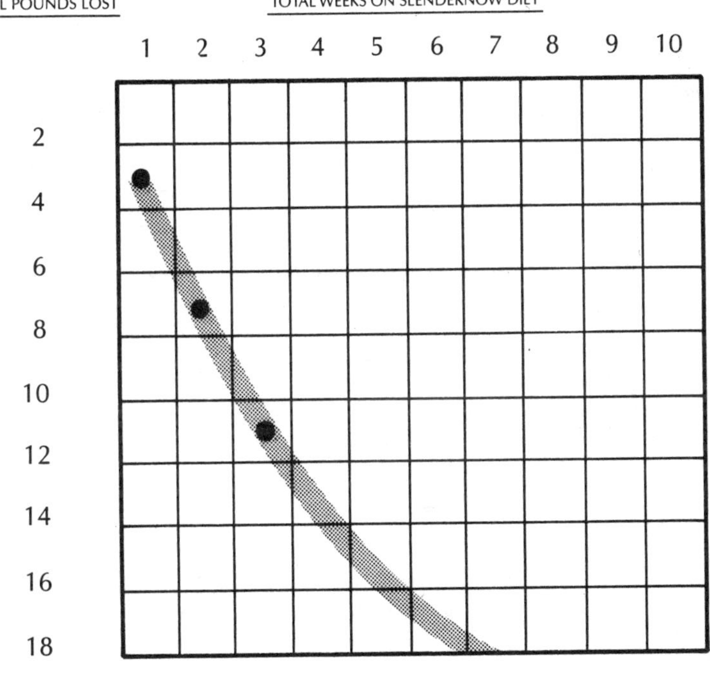

TABLE 6.2

Inches Lost Progress Toward Goal

		WEEKS ON SLENDERNOW DIET				
MEASUREMENT	START	2	4	6	8	GOAL
Waist	____	__	__	__	__	____
Neck	____	__	__	__	__	____
Chest or Bust	____	__	__	__	__	____
Arm	____	__	__	__	__	____
Hips	____	__	__	__	__	____
Thighs	____	__	__	__	__	____
Calf	____	__	__	__	__	____
Ankle	____	__	__	__	__	____
Women's Dress Size	____	__	__	__	__	____

Note: Exercise may "build up" certain areas. As you lose fat and build your figure and strength, weight is redistributed. Always measure at the same spot.

TABLE 6.3

FLAB LOSS PROGRESS

AREA	WEEKS ON SLENDERNOW DIET					
	0	2	4	6	8	10
Waist	__	__	__	__	__	__
Chest	__	__	__	__	__	__
Arms	__	__	__	__	__	__
Thighs	__	__	__	__	__	__

Place a minus sign (−) in the appropriate box if the body area is mostly flabby. Place a zero (0) in the box if the body area has a firm base covered with some flab. Place a plus sign (+) in the box if the body area has become firm.

It's hard to see the changes from day to day. You may suddenly become aware that your clothes fit better, but the change was gradual. You may even forget how overweight you were and how tight your clothes fit. The records will help keep you encouraged as you progress. The numbers will impress you.

Diet Tables

I do not recommend diet tables for several reasons. Most people use them as evidence that they are obviously "large-boned" or "large-framed." And, of course, there are our humorous friends who will look at them and pronounce that they are too short for their weight.

My point is that there are several body types and different degrees of muscularity. A well-muscled athlete can weigh much more than suggested by the weight tables and not have excess fat. On the other hand, a poorly conditioned person can be in the desired weight range, but still have a potbelly. It's fat we are interested in, not bone and muscle.

Presently, there is controversy about the importance of the weight tables. They are being adjusted upward to reflect the results of recent studies that indicate that people live longer if they are a little heavier than the desirable weights listed in the old tables.

My personal opinion is that this research primarily shows that proper nourishment leads to a longer life span than malnourishment. Unfortunately, most people today have achieved fashionable thinness not by burning calories with healthy activity, but by living on diet sodas and eating too little food. Thus, they lack the nutrients necessary to maintain health and resist disease.

You can have it both ways. You can be slender and well nourished. A more detailed study would undoubtedly find that a well-nourished person having a firm, trim and conditioned body will be healthier and live longer than any other category of persons.

Pictures Tell the Story

Your biggest booster of all may be to take "before" and "after" photos. Take a shot of yourself in a relaxed pose in a bathing suit or shorts and T-shirt. Write your weight and the date on the back and tape the photo on your refrigerator. This will help keep you from nibbling. Take it with you when you weigh and measure yourself. Look in the mirror and compare.

Now, before you read on, make those "starting" measurements before they disappear. These records will become your source of pride in the weeks ahead.

7

Okay, so you're ready to begin! Yet proper preparation is required for success. If you start on the spur of the moment, you may increase your risk of quitting on the spur of the moment because you didn't have the right foods or were tempted by leftovers in the refrigerator.

Supplies

First, you should get your supplies together. You will need protein powder, polyunsaturated oil, skim milk, juice, flavorings, sweeteners, vitamin pills, and a mixer. Since you are probably going to save $75 or so a month with the milkshake meals, you may wish to invest part of that savings in a blender. Blenders are, of course, handy even when your diet is over.

The specifications for the protein powder and polyunsaturated oil are given in Chapter 9. The specifications for the vitamins are given in Chapter 11.

You should also round up measuring spoons (teaspoon, half-teaspoon and tablespoon) and a measuring cup. You will be able to estimate the proper amounts without measuring, but let's get started correctly. It's a good idea to keep a diet notebook too. A notebook not only helps you keep track of your progress, but it helps you learn and overcome your bad eating habits.

For the next three days, keep a record of what you eat and why you ate. You will be surprised at how many calories you usually eat and that you weren't always hungry when you ate. Sometimes you eat because you've just arrived home or wanted something to snack on while watching TV just out of habit. You will find this information useful when you learn better eating habits before going off the Slendernow Diet Program.

CHECKLIST

- ___ Doctor's OK
- ___ Starting measurements taken
- ___ Protein powder
- ___ Polyunsaturated oil
- ___ Flavorings
- ___ Sweeteners
- ___ Mixer or blender
- ___ Measuring cup and spoons
- ___ Vitamin pills
- ___ Skim milk
- ___ Juice
- ___ Notebook
- ___ Food for main meal menus

You should choose your menus for the first week and then purchase the necessary items. Shop with a list to prevent impulse buying. If you are going to eat foods different from the rest of the family, place them in a brown bag in the refrigerator and tell everyone that they are "hands off."

Warm-Up Period

Best results are obtained when you prepare yourself mentally as well. Don't plunge right in. Get used to the milkshakes and new eating habits gradually. The following three-day plan lets you make the transition smoothly.

WARM-UP DAY 1

Get rid of the empty calorie junk foods lying around the house. Give them away, throw them away or even go on a binge and eat them up. But get rid of them by the end of warm-up day one.

Exercise very lightly. Bend a lot, stretch a lot, and take a brisk ten-minute walk.

Drink a glass of water at midmorning and midafternoon. Take a vitamin pill.

WARM-UP DAY 2

At breakfast, drink a Diet Shake made with one tablespoon of protein powder instead of two tablespoons of protein powder, and omit the oil. Drink this before your regular breakfast. Stop eating your regular breakfast when you feel full.

Eat no sweets or junk food. Drink a glass of water at midmorning and midafternoon. Don't forget to take your vitamin pill. Exercise lightly by bending, stretching, and doing a couple of sit-ups and push-ups. Take a brisk ten-minute walk.

WARM-UP DAY 3

Replace your usual breakfast with a regular Diet Shake. Take your vitamin pill at breakfast.

If you are hungry at midmorning, you should drink a glass of water and enjoy a small snack of *one* of the following:

- five chewable protein tablets
- 1 slice of cheese
- 1 hard-boiled egg
- 1 fresh fruit
- 1 cup unsalted, unbuttered popcorn
- unlimited celery or carrot sticks

Exercise lightly as on Warm-Up Day Two.

Now you're ready to begin the Slendernow Diet Program, and you will be successful.

8

The Slendernow Diet is not only convenient, it is simple. There are only a few rules to follow. The program is flexible to meet your needs.

The only rules that you have to remember are:

- Never skip a meal
- Eat one main meal every day (the only exception is that you can eat only the three Diet Shake meals once or twice during a plateau period)
- Be sure to add the oil
- Do not let more than 4–5 hours pass between meals
- Exercise 10–20 minutes, four times a week

Table 8.1 lists the daily activity schedule "required" for the Slendernow Diet Program.

TABLE 8.1

Daily Activity

TIME	ACTIVITY
On Arising	10 sit-ups
Breakfast	Diet Shake
	Vitamin pill
Midmorning	Glass of water
Lunch	Diet Shake or Main Meal
Midafternoon	Glass of water
Dinner	Main Meal (or Diet Shake if main meal has already been eaten)
Midevening	Exercise period (10–12 minutes, 4 days/week)

In the previous chapters, I have discussed the nutritional aspects of the Slendernow Diet Program. While it is true that you can lose weight by diet alone, exercising improves your health, improves your figure, and helps you safely lose weight at a faster rate. It is a definite part of the "total" Slendernow Diet Program and should become a regular part of your life.

The exercises of the Slendernow Diet are 10 sit-ups daily, and four 10–12 minute aerobic-type exercise periods each week. The aerobic exercises include any two of the following: walking briskly, rebounding, jogging, biking, jumping rope, or dancing. I recommend that you choose two exercises and alternate them. My recommendations are walking briskly and rebounding. Rebounding is jogging in place on a springy platform. It's fun and it's easy on your bones. Choose the two exercises that are the most pleasurable for you. Chapter 12 will discuss exercising more fully.

The Slendernow Diet Program also involves reexamining your eating habits. You will learn several tricks that will help you stay slender. Scientists like to call this behavior modification, but it is only learning how to enjoy staying slender. You are the sum of your habits. This will be discussed in Chapter 13.

That's all there is to the daily plan. Uncomplicated, isn't it? It will blend in with your present lifestyle as you lose weight, and by the end of eight weeks, you will have improved your lifestyle—without much conscious effort—to maintain your figure.

The Slendernow Diet Program is simple, but don't try to "outsmart" it! Every aspect of the program is designed the way it is deliberately.

- Don't skip a milkshake. You will get hungry.
- Don't hold back on the oil in the belief you will save a few calories. You'll miss vital nutrients and become hungry after 3½ hours. The Diet Shakes are designed to control hunger 4½ to 5 hours.
- Don't cut back on meals unless you are not losing weight at the suggested rate.

Okay, let's begin. Select your favorite Diet Shake flavors in the next chapter.

9

Warning—diet milkshakes and juice-shakes are habit forming. That's because they taste so good and are so easy to prepare. This chapter could be called, "The Joys of Not Cooking!"

The Diet Shakes do more than just taste good. They supply variety to keep the Slendernow Diet interesting. They are convenient and inexpensive to prepare. But most important, they insure a balanced, nutritious meal of controlled, measured amounts of foods. Thus, there is no under- or overeating or calorie counting. The 10 to 15 percent error common in calorie counting due to disguised calories alone often sabotages conventional diets. The Diet Shakes overcome this error.

The "meat" (pun intended) of the Diet Shake is powdered protein. You can make the protein powder yourself by mixing equal parts of powdered egg whites and dried milk. However, the commercial protein powders made largely from soybean protein mix more easily with milk or juice and produce a much more palatable Diet Shake. Commercial protein powders are well worth their cost. Modern protein powders mix smoothly by shaking or stirring alone and stay smoothly mixed longer than the original protein powders. Modern protein powders also are usually fortified with vitamins and minerals to improve their nourishment.

Diet Shakes are truly inexpensive. The Slendernow Diet usually saves dieters $75 to $100 each month. Some of this saving is a result of less food being required for the diet, and some is attributed to the convenience of Diet Shakes, which reduce the need to eat out. However, the Diet Shake saves money even on the Slendernow Maintenance Program. A balanced-nutrition meal-in-a-glass is just less expensive than a balanced-nutrition conventional meal.

Admittedly, a so-called breakfast of a cup of coffee and a

cigarette is less expensive than a Diet Shake. However, we must compare like to like. What is the cost of your favorite nutritionally balanced breakfast or lunch (disregard wasted leftovers and preparation costs)? Now add together the cost of a 22-ounce can of powdered protein, two gallons of skim milk, and a pint of polyunsaturated oil. Divide this figure by thirty-one to find the per-serving cost. Quite a bargain, isn't it?

There are several formulations of protein powder commercially available. Some have no carbohydrate; these are designed for the low-carbohydrate diets that produce ketosis. Although the exact percentage of protein, carbohydrate and fat contained in the protein powder is not critical, I have found the best palatability and mixing qualities to be a powder approximately 80 percent protein, 10 percent carbohydrate and the remainder mineral ash and fat.

The carbohydrate content should include some bran and fruit-sugar (fructose) or milk-sugar (lactose). The protein can be largely soybean protein, but some milk protein (casein, nonfat milk solids, or casinates) should be included. Since most of the commercial Diet Shakes contain milk, additional milk is not critical, and the shakes can easily be made with juice.

If the milk protein in the commercial powders is troublesome (if you are allergic to milk, for example) use egg whites with the juice-shake recipes. For those who have lactose intolerance, the small amount of lactose in most protein powders is insignificant, but you can use the egg-white powder with juice or add the enzyme lactase to the milkshake to digest the milk sugar for you. Still, I believe your best option is to use the commercial protein powders and add one to two tablespoons of cream plus fruit juice.

In summary, the Diet Shakes offer the following advantages:

1. They are safe.
2. They provide less opportunity to cheat on food proportions.
3. They can be prepared rapidly.
4. They provide adequate protein.
5. There are many delicious variations.
6. They cost less than coffee and doughnuts.
7. Each Diet Shake is a complete meal.

Oil

The Slendernow Diet requires that polyunsaturated oil be added to the Diet Shakes for several reasons. First of all, the polyunsaturated oil—linoleic acid—is essential for health. We must be extra sure to get enough when we restrict our food intake. Second, fats and oils help to absorb the fat-soluble vitamins A, D, E, and K that we need for health. Third, we need fat or oil in the meal to prevent hunger that otherwise would occur after three to four hours. Fats and oils digest more slowly than carbohydrates and protein, and, as they digest, they maintain the proper blood sugar level to prevent hunger.

A fourth reason is that there is substantial evidence that polyunsaturated oils aid in the process that "burns" stored body fat. This evidence is not conclusive and is thus subject to debate. However, the finding is that the fatter people are, the less polyunsaturated fatty acid they have in their bodies, and vice versa (P. Oster, et al., *Research in Experimental Medicine,* 175:287–291, 1979).

A fifth purpose in adding the oil is that it aids in maintaining regularity. Oil also adds a "creamier" feeling to the Diet Shakes.

You have two options for adding the polyunsaturated oil to your Diet Shakes. The preferred choice is to add one tablespoon of polyunsaturated oil to your morning Diet Shake. This is the most convenient and it fuels your body before you need extra energy. The second choice is to use one-half tablespoon in each Diet Shake.

The polyunsaturated oil can be safflower oil, sunflower oil, wheat germ oil, corn oil, rice oil, or soybean oil. A mixture provides a better nutritional balance. An excellent blend is equal parts corn oil, rice oil, soybean oil, and safflower oil. Since polyunsaturated oil requires vitamin E to function properly in the body, it is wise to add vitamin E as a natural preservative to the oil and to make sure there is adequate vitamin E in your vitamin supplement. Some oils have had their natural vitamin E removed to provide a source of the vitamin for dietary supplements. If an oil smells or tastes rancid—throw it out. Refrigerate the oil once you've opened the container.

By the way, don't worry about the Shakes tasting oily. You won't taste it.

In review, polyunsaturated oil is required for the following reasons:

1. It's essential for health.
2. It helps absorb fat-soluble vitamins A, D, E, and K.
3. Prevents hunger 3 to 4 hours after taking it.
4. Aids in burning body fat.
5. Maintains regularity.
6. Imparts a "creaminess" to the shakes.
7. Improves skin and hair.

Milk

Skim (nonfat) milk is preferred for the Diet Shakes because you can also use it with your main meal. If you don't like the taste of skim milk with your meal, start out with milk containing 2 percent fat, then use milk with 1 percent fat and *then* go to nonfat skim milk.

Flavors

Baking extracts are excellent flavorings for your Diet Shakes. They can be found in supermarkets and some health food and drugstores. Flavored syrups can also be used, but keep in mind that their sugars contain extra calories.

Tips on Preparing Slendernow Diet Shakes

It is important to have variety in your shakes as you do in your regular meals. This is an eating regimen and it is important that you enjoy it.

The protein powder mixes well enough in milk or juice so that a blender is really not needed, unless fruit you want to mix with is whole. When mixing the shake in a blender, start blender at low speed first with the juice or milk only. Slowly add the powder and increase speed. Fruit or flavoring may then be added. Add ice (4–6 cubes) last and then turn blender to full speed for about 20 seconds.

For best digestive results, take your shake within 30 minutes from the time you wake up in the morning.

Adding a raw egg to your shake will not only provide additional quality calories for those who desire more, but it will also make the shake much smoother.

Do not gulp the shake down. Consume it slowly as you would a hot cup of coffee. This will greatly aid in proper digestion.

The shake can be made at nighttime and then frozen in a thermos bottle to be taken to work for lunch the next day. Shake well before drinking.

One tablespoon of lemon juice will eliminate the slight grainy taste, if you discover it.

The Diet Shakes also can be served hot. Heat (do not boil) the milk before mixing. Or the Diet Shakes can be "thickened" by placing them in the freezer after mixing for 15–20 minutes and then restirring or blending for 5–10 seconds.

Diet Shake Recipes

Use your imagination to design delightful flavors to suit your taste preference, but here are 101 recipes to get you started.

There are four main classes of Diet Shakes; protein milkshakes, protein juice-shakes, combination milk and juice shakes, and miscellaneous. The juice-shakes taste like sherbets and the milkshakes taste like ice cream milkshakes.

Milkshakes

The general formula for the following protein milkshakes is as follows:

8 fluid ounces (1 cup) of skim milk
2 rounded tablespoons of protein powder
Polyunsaturated oil (0, ½, 1 tablespoon depending on how you decide to distribute your daily allotment)
4–6 ice cubes (if blender is used)
Sweetener (1 package of sugar substitute, or ½ to 1 teaspoon of honey or fructose) if desired

The above ingredients are the Basic Mix referred to in the following Diet Shake recipes. The Juice Mix is the same, except the milk is omitted.

VANILLA FLAVORS

1. Vanilla
Basic Mix
1 teaspoon vanilla extract

2. Vanilla Butternut
Basic Mix
1 teaspoon vanilla extract
½–1 teaspoon butter and nut extract
dash of cinnamon

CHOCOLATE FLAVORS

3. Milk Chocolate
Basic Mix
1 teaspoon chocolate extract
1 teaspoon vanilla extract optional

4. Double Chocolate
Basic Mix (but use low-fat chocolate milk instead of skim milk)
1 teaspoon chocolate extract

5. Fudgesicle
Basic Mix (but use low-fat chocolate milk instead of skim milk)
10 ice cubes (rather than 4–6)

6. Chocolate Mint
Basic Mix
1 teaspoon chocolate extract
½–1 teaspoon peppermint extract

7. Black Forest
Basic Mix
½ teaspoon chocolate extract
½ teaspoon black walnut extract

8. Rum Chocolate
Basic Mix
1 teaspoon chocolate extract
1 teaspoon mint extract
1 teaspoon rum extract

9. Tip of Angels' Wings
Basic Mix
1 teaspoon chocolate extract
1 teaspoon brandy extract

10. Caledonia
Basic Mix
1 teaspoon chocolate extract
1 teaspoon brandy extract
sprinkle with cinnamon

11. Capri
Basic Mix
1 teaspoon chocolate extract
1 teaspoon brandy extract
1 teaspoon banana extract

12. Banshee
Basic Mix
1 teaspoon chocolate extract
½–1 teaspoon banana extract

13. Choco-maple
Basic Mix
½–1 teaspoon chocolate extract
½ teaspoon maple extract

14. Choco-mocha
Basic Mix
1 teaspoon chocolate extract
½ teaspoon decaffeinated instant coffee

15. Choco-mocha mint
Basic Mix
1 teaspoon chocolate extract
½ teaspoon decaffeinated instant coffee
½ teaspoon peppermint extract

16. Almond Joy Shake
Basic Mix
½ teaspoon chocolate extract
½ teaspoon coconut extract
½ teaspoon almond extract

17. Chocolate Peanut Butter
Basic Mix
1 teaspoon chocolate extract
½–1 teaspoon peanut butter

COFFEE FLAVORS

18. Coffee Shake
Basic Mix
1–2 teaspoons decaffeinated instant coffee

19. Coffee Mint
Basic Mix
2 teaspoons decaffeinated instant coffee
½ teaspoon peppermint extract

20. Mocha Shake

Basic Mix
2 teaspoons decaffeinated instant coffee
1 teaspoon chocolate extract

21. Mocha Mint

Basic Mix
2 teaspoons decaffeinated instant coffee
1 teaspoon chocolate extract
½ teaspoon peppermint extract

22. Algeria

Basic Mix
2 teaspoons decaffeinated instant coffee
1 teaspoon rum extract

23. Black Magic

Basic Mix
2 teaspoons decaffeinated instant coffee
1 teaspoon rum extract
1 teaspoon cinnamon

24. Cara Sposa

Basic Mix
2 teaspoons decaffeinated instant coffee
1 teaspoon brandy extract

25. Irish Coffee Shake

Basic Mix
2 teaspoons decaffeinated instant coffee
1 teaspoon brandy extract
1 teaspoon rum extract
1 teaspoon marshmallow whip

(also see Choco-mocha (14) and Choco-mocha mint (15) shakes)

BANANA FLAVORS

26. Banana Shake

Basic Mix
1 teaspoon banana extract
½ teaspoon vanilla extract

27. Real Banana

Basic Mix
1 sliced banana
½ teaspoon vanilla extract

28. Double Banana

Basic Mix
1 sliced banana
½ teaspoon banana extract
1 teaspoon vanilla extract

29. Florida Cooler

Basic Mix
½ teaspoon banana extract
½ teaspoon pineapple extract
sprinkle with nutmeg

(also see Capri (11), Caribbean Champagne (95), Golden Boston (65), Banshee (12), Island Champagne (94), and Panana (63) combination shakes)

OTHER EXCITING FLAVORS

30. Blackberry Shake

Basic Mix
1 teaspoon blackberry extract or fresh blackberries

31. Brandy Alexander

Basic Mix
1 teaspoon brandy extract

32. Brandy Alexander's Sister

Basic Mix
1 teaspoon brandy extract
½ teaspoon peppermint extract

33. Butter Almond

Basic Mix
1 teaspoon butter almond extract

34. Butter Rum

Basic Mix
1 teaspoon butter rum extract
1 teaspoon vanilla extract (optional)

35. Butterscotch

Basic Mix
1 teaspoon butterscotch extract
1 teaspoon vanilla extract

36. Cherry Shake

Basic Mix
1 teaspoon cherry extract or 5–6 cherries

37. Cherry Flip

Basic Mix
1 teaspoon cherry extract or 5–6 cherries

1 teaspoon rum or brandy extract
sprinkle of nutmeg

also see Cherry Fizz (93 shake)

38. Egglicious

Basic Mix
1–2 raw eggs (shells included)
1 teaspoon vanilla extract

39. Orange Blossom

Basic Mix
½ teaspoon orange extract
½ teaspoon brandy extract

40. Creamsicle

Basic Mix
½ teaspoon orange extract
½ teaspoon vanilla extract

41. Peach Shake

Basic Mix
1 peach or 1 teaspoon peach extract
1 teaspoon vanilla extract

42. Pineapple Shake

Basic Mix
1 teaspoon pineapple extract

43. Shave Tail

Basic Mix
1 teaspoon pineapple extract
½ teaspoon peppermint extract

44. Piña Colada

Basic Mix
1 teaspoon rum extract
1 teaspoon pineapple extract
1 teaspoon coconut extract

45. Real Piña Colada

Juice Mix
½ cup crushed pineapple
2 oz. skim milk
4 oz. Diet 7-Up or club soda
½ teaspoon coconut extract
½ teaspoon vanilla extract or rum extract

46. Little Colada

Basic Mix
½ teaspoon rum extract
½ teaspoon coconut extract

47. Plum Smooth

Basic Mix
6 plums
1 banana
1 teaspoon vanilla extract

48. Raspberry Shake

Basic Mix
1 teaspoon raspberry extract or fresh fruit

49. Rum Daisy

Basic Mix
1 teaspoon raspberry mix
1 teaspoon rum extract

50. Strawberry Shake

Basic Mix
1 teaspoon strawberry extract or 4 strawberries
1 teaspoon vanilla extract

51. Yogurt Shake

Basic Mix
2–4 oz. favorite flavor yogurt

52. Health Shake

Basic Mix
1 teaspoon powdered liver
1 teaspoon lecithin

53. Energy Shake

Basic Mix
1 teaspoon powdered liver
1 teaspoon yeast

54. Nirvana

Basic Mix
1 teaspoon powdered liver
1 teaspoon yeast
1 teaspoon lecithin

55. Jell-o Sherbet

Juice Mix
½ cup half-set dietetic gelatin
4 oz. fruit juice

56. Jell-o Shake

Basic Mix
½ cup hardened dietetic gelatin (Jell-o)

COMBINATION SHAKES

The following are smooth blends tastefully combining milk and fruit juice, set off with a touch of contrasting flavoring.

57. Shirley Temple

Juice Mix
4 oz. skim milk
4 oz. orange juice
1 tablespoon lemon juice
1 teaspoon cherry extract

58. La Jolla

Juice Mix
4 oz. skim milk
2 oz. orange juice
1 tablespoon lemon juice
½ teaspoon banana extract

59. Creamed Orange
Juice Mix
3 oz. skim milk
3 oz. orange juice
1 teaspoon sherry extract

60. Triple Fruit Cooler
Juice Mix
2 oz. skim milk
6 oz. orange juice
4 strawberries
½ teaspoon banana or pineapple extract

61. Soda Floats
Juice Mix
5 oz. skim milk
3 oz. diet soda
(root beer and black cherry are the best flavors)

62. Apple Pie
Juice Mix
6 oz. skim milk
2 oz. apple juice
1 teaspoon lemon juice
cinnamon and nutmeg

63. Panana
Juice Mix
4 oz. skim milk
4 oz. papaya juice
1 sliced banana or 1 teaspoon banana extract

JUICE SHAKES

The following are delicious summer coolers having the flavor of sherbets:

64. O.J. Shake
Juice Mix
6–8 oz. orange juice

65. Golden Boston
Juice Mix
6 oz. orange juice
½–1 teaspoon banana extract

66. Sun Shake
Juice Mix
4 oz. orange juice
1 banana
1 tablespoon lecithin
(vitamin C powder optional)

67. Knickerbocker
Juice Mix
6 oz. orange juice
1 teaspoon lemon juice
1 teaspoon raspberry extract
1 teaspoon rum extract

68. Borinquen
Juice Mix
3 oz. orange juice
3 oz. lime juice
1 teaspoon rum extract
2 strawberries (or 1 teaspoon pineapple extract)

69. Honolulu Fizz
Juice Mix
4 oz. orange juice
2 oz. Diet 7-Up
½ teaspoon pineapple juice
½ teaspoon lemon juice

70. Punchy Brandy
Juice Mix
3 oz. orange juice
4 oz. weak tea
1 oz. lemon juice
1 teaspoon brandy extract

71. Fruit Salute
Juice Mix
4 oz. orange juice
4 oz. water
1 tablespoon lemon juice
1 teaspoon pineapple extract
1 teaspoon rum extract

72. Strawberry-Orange
Juice Mix
4 oz. orange juice
4 strawberries or 1 teaspoon strawberry extract

73. Tropical Strawberry-Orange
Juice Mix
6 oz. orange juice
4 strawberries or 1 teaspoon strawberry extract
½ teaspoon pineapple extract

74. Apple Jack
Juice Mix
6 oz. apple juice or sliced apple with water
Juice of 1 lemon

75. Daisy Star
Juice Mix
6 oz. apple juice or sliced apple with water
1 teaspoon raspberry extract
1 teaspoon lemon juice

76. Apple Fizz
Juice Mix
4 oz. apple juice
2 oz. Diet 7-Up

1 teaspoon brandy extract

(also see Apple Pie (62) shake)

77. Carrot Shake

Juice Mix
6 oz. carrot juice

78. V.J. Shake

Juice Mix
6 oz. mixed vegetable juice (V-8)

79. Cranapple Shake

Juice Mix
6 oz. cranapple juice

80. Cranberry

Juice Mix
6 oz. cranberry juice

81. Cape Codder

Juice Mix
5 oz. cranberry juice
1 oz. lime juice
1 teaspoon rum extract

82. Grape Shake

Juice Mix
6 oz. grape juice or 25 grapes with water

83. Purple Martin

Juice Mix
4 oz. grape juice
2 oz. Diet 7-Up
1 teaspoon bran

84. Grapefruit

Juice Mix
6 oz. grapefruit juice

85. Minty Grapefruit

Juice Mix
6 oz. grapefruit juice
½ teaspoon peppermint extract

86. Nevada Cocktail

Juice Mix
6 oz. grapefruit juice
1 tablespoon lemon juice
1 teaspoon rum extract

87. Hawaiian Punch

Juice Mix
6 oz. diet Hawaiian Punch
1 teaspoon lemon juice

88. Melonade

Juice Mix
1 cup cubed watermelon (seeded)
2 oz. club soda or Diet 7-Up
½ teaspoon lemon juice
Mint leaf garnish

89. Cantaloupade

Juice Mix
4 tablespoons cantaloupe
2 oz. Diet 7-Up
dash of lemon juice

90. Papaya Supreme

Juice Mix
1 cubed papaya
½ nectarine
2 strawberries
3 grapes
½ teaspoon lime juice
dash of ginger

91. Tomato Spice

Juice Mix
6–8 oz. tomato juice
½ tablespoon lemon juice
¼ tablespoon Worcestershire sauce
(drop of hot sauce optional)
dash salt and pepper

92. Pizza Shake

Juice Mix
6–8 oz. tomato juice
½ teaspoon oregano
dash pepper

MISCELLANEOUS FIZZES AND FOODS

Sparkle can be added by using club soda or Diet 7-Up as a source of carbonation. Soups and puddings are also pleasant variations.

93. Cherry Fizz

Juice Mix
8 oz. Diet 7-Up
1 teaspoon cherry extract
1 teaspoon lemon juice
1 teaspoon brandy extract

94. Island Champagne

Juice Mix
8 oz. Diet 7-Up
1 teaspoon banana extract

95. Caribbean Champagne

Juice Mix
8 oz. Diet 7-Up
1 teaspoon rum extract
1 teaspoon banana extract
½ teaspoon pineapple extract

96. Tropical Lemonade

Juice Mix
6 oz. Diet 7-Up
1 oz. lemon juice
1 oz. lime juice

97. Hudson Bay

Juice Mix
6 oz. Diet 7-Up
2 oz. orange juice
1 teaspoon cherry extract
1 teaspoon lime juice
1 teaspoon rum extract

98. Pineapple Fizz

Juice Mix
8 oz. Diet 7-Up
1 tablespoon lemon juice
1 teaspoon pineapple extract

99. Cocomacque

Juice Mix
5 oz. Diet 7-Up
2 oz. orange juice
1 oz. lime juice
1 teaspoon pineapple extract

100. Soup

6 oz. bouillion (chicken or beef) or vegetable juice or tomato juice
Heat, then add Juice Mix
Thicken, if desired, with ½ teaspoon cornstarch

101. Chocolate Pudding

Juice Mix
1 pkg. unflavored gelatin
¼ c. boiling water
⅓ c. powdered milk (2% low-fat dry milk)
4 or 5 pkg. artificial sweetener (to equal 8–10 tsp. sugar)
1½ teaspoon unsweetened carob powder or 1½ teaspoon chocolate extract
(Optional: 1 teaspoon rum extract and 1 teaspoon decaffeinated coffee.)

Pour cold water and gelatin into blender. While blender is running, add boiling water, milk, sweetener, Juice Mix, carob, and all extracts. Add ice cubes, one at a time, until thick.

10

The Slendernow Diet main meal serves several purposes besides the simple joy of eating. The main meal provides you with an opportunity to eat with family, friends, or business colleagues without broadcasting that you are dieting. The main meal also supplies ample calories so that you don't lose weight too fast and risk metabolizing your own lean tissue. However, the most important function of the main meal is to balance the diet by supplying generous quantities of vitamins, minerals, and complex carbohydrates.

The main meals include servings from four basic food groups. It is possible that not all of our essential nutrients have been identified yet, so you should eat a wide variety of foods to be sure you are not excluding something you need. In fact, that sums up our entire wisdom about eating—eat a diversified diet and eat in moderation.

Enjoy as many different main meals as you can. This will keep your diet interesting. Boredom and hunger are the biggest threats to a diet program. Vary the flavor of your Diet Shakes—even if you have to give up your favorite flavor for a day—and vary your main meals.

There are 34 main-meal menus given here as suggestions. You don't have to follow them as you can plan your own menus. I highly recommend that you partake of at least ten different menus. If you are adventurous, you may wish to try 20 or 30 different menus.

Three of the menus are vegetarian, but vegetarians can include some of their favorites so as to have ten main-meal menus. There are not that many overweight vegetarians, but there are more than many vegetarians realize. Whenever I lecture on dieting, I usually have one or two questions from overweight vegetarians. Often they are slow-metabolizers or hypoglycemic. Some are omnivores who have recently switched to vegetarianism but haven't lost their extra pounds.

Some menus are designed especially for ethnic or regional palates. After all, this is truly an All-American diet. Other menus are designed for picnic and hot- or cold-weather eating. Choose your favorites and dig in.

The Slendernow Diet main meals are designed with the "FLAB" (Fat Liquidating Ability Barometer) concept that I developed in 1979.* The FLAB concept helps design meals that are balanced in terms of protein, carbohydrate, and fat so that the foods digest evenly and contribute their nourishment to the bloodstream at a controlled pace. This even control minimizes the need for insulin and thus minimizes fat-production and encourages fat-burning.

The Slendernow Diet main meals are designed at 600, 750, and 1050 calorie levels. The 600-calorie meals are for the individual who is a slow metabolizer and cannot lose weight above 1,000 calories per day. The 600-calorie meals can also be used by crash dieters who insist on losing weight as fast as possible rather than at the optimal rate recommended. I recognize that occasionally there are special needs in the everyday world where someone must lose weight quickly in spite of the hardship put on their bodies. Actors and athletes sometimes must meet weight limits or not make the cast or team. If someone is going to crash diet, I would rather that they do it as safely as possible. The 600-calorie meals provide adequate nourishment.

The Slendernow Diet 750-calorie main meals are for women and provide 1,200 calories total intake per day. The 1050-calorie main meals will provide 1500 calories daily for men. Under no circumstances should anyone eat more than he feels comfortable with. You should not eat after you feel full. You should never feel "stuffed."

The 750-calorie main meals average 40 to 70 grams of protein, 55 to 90 grams of carbohydrate, and 15 to 30 grams of fat. A typical 750-calorie main meal would be 57 grams of protein, 80 grams of carbohydrate and 23 grams of fat.

*Passwater, R. A., *Nutritional Perspectives*, 2(1) 32–45 (January 1979).

As mentioned in the first chapter, you can choose to eat your main meal either at lunch or at dinner. Studies have shown that food eaten earlier in the day tends to be converted directly into energy for our daily activity, whereas the same calorie level of food eaten after our main energy requirement is over tends to be converted to body fat. In other words, we should put fuel into the body before we need its energy, not afterwards when the food energy will not be used and is thus stored as fat. Therefore, scientifically speaking, it is preferable to eat the main meal at lunch. However, human considerations are more important than scientific factors.

If you prefer to plan your own main meals, turn to Chapter 15 and review the section on the basic four food groups. Use the calorie counter in the appendix to keep the menu within the targeted range.

If you use the suggested menus, you may also wish to use the "good old-fashioned" recipes that follow the menus. Of course, you may use your own recipes if you wish.

Main Meal Menu Index

Beef	5, 8, 10–13, 15, 17, 19, 21, 22, 28–30
Fast Foods	11, 16, 18
Fish	1, 7, 14, 16, 24–27
Ham	9
Lamb Chop	2
Liver	4, 23
Poultry	3, 6, 18
Italian (spaghetti, lasagna, pizza)	20, 30, 34
Vegetarian	31–33

MAIN MEAL No. 1

(Recipes 1–8)

FOOD	PORTIONS PER CALORIE TOTAL		
	600	750	1050
Tossed salad with	1½ c	1½ c	1½ c
salad dressing	1 T	1 T	1 T
Fillet of flounder	4 oz	5 oz	8 oz
Mashed potato with butter	1 c	1½ c	1½ c
Corn, canned	½ c	¾ c	¾ c
Whole wheat bread with butter	1 sl	1 sl	2 sl
Skim milk	8 oz	10 oz	12 oz

MAIN MEAL No. 2

(Recipes 1–7, 9–11)

FOOD	PORTIONS PER CALORIE TOTAL		
	600	750	1050
Tossed salad with	1½ c	1½ c	1½ c
salad dressing	1 T	1 T	1 T
Rib lamb chop, broiled	3 oz	4 oz	6 oz
Rice	½ c	½ c	1 c
Whole grain bread			
(or bran muffin)	1	2	1
butter	1 t	1 t	1 t
Skim milk	8 oz	10 oz	12 oz

MAIN MEAL No. 3

(Recipes 12–16)

FOOD	PORTIONS PER CALORIE TOTAL		
	600	750	1050
Fruit cocktail	1 c	1½ c	2 c
Roast turkey	5 oz	6 oz	9 oz
stuffing	¼ c	¼ c	½ c
Sweet potato, baked or stuffed	½	1	1
butter	1 t	1 t	1 t
Asparagus, creamed	4 spears	5 spears	6 spears
Tomato	3 sl	4 sl	6 sl
Whole grain bread	1 sl	1 sl	2 sl
butter	1 t	1 t	2 t
Skim milk	8 oz	10 oz	12 oz

MAIN MEAL No. 4

(Recipes 1–7, 11, 16, 17, 18)

FOOD	PORTIONS PER CALORIE TOTAL		
	600	750	1050
Salad	1½ c	1½ c	1½ c
dressing	1 T	1 T	1 T
Broiled calves' liver	4 oz	5 oz	8 oz
Onions, sliced	⅓ c	½ c	⅔ c
Sweet potato, baked or stuffed	½	1	1
Corn bread or bran muffin	1 sl	1 sl	2 sl
butter	1 t	1 t	2 t
Skim milk	8 oz	10 oz	12 oz

MAIN MEAL No. 5

(Recipes 1–7, 19, 20)

FOOD	PORTIONS PER CALORIE TOTAL		
	600	750	1050
Tossed salad	1½ c	1½ c	1½ c
dressing	1 t	1 t	1 t
Sirloin strip steak, broiled	4 oz	5 oz	8 oz
Baked potato	½	1	1
(or macaroni salad)			
butter	1 t	1 t	1 t
Beets with greens	½ c	1 c	1½ c
or beets in orange sauce			
Whole wheat bread	1 sl	1 sl	2 sl
butter	1 t	1 t	2 t
Skim milk	8 oz	10 oz	12 oz

MAIN MEAL No. 6

(Recipes 1–7, 21, 22)

FOOD	PORTIONS PER CALORIE TOTAL		
	600	750	1050
Tossed salad	1½ c	1½ c	1½ c
dressing	1 T	1 T	1 T
Roasted chicken	5 oz	6 oz	9 oz
Baked potato or potato salad	½	1	1
butter	1 t	1 t	1 t
Green beans	½ c	1 c	1 c
Whole grain bread (or bran muffin)	1 sl	1 sl	2 sl
butter	1 t	1 t	2 t
Skim milk	8 oz	10 oz	12 oz

MAIN MEAL No. 7

(Recipes 1–7, 8, 10, 11)

FOOD	PORTIONS PER CALORIE TOTAL		
	600	750	1050
Salad	1½ c	1½ c	1½ c
dressing	1 T	1 T	1 T
Broiled red snapper	6 oz	7 oz	9 oz
butter	1 t	1 t	1 t
Rice	½ c	1 c	1½ c
Beets (diced) (or summer squash or soybeans sprouts)	½ c	1 c	1 c
Whole grain bread or muffin	1 sl	1 sl	2 sl
butter	1 t	1 t	2 t
Skim milk	8 oz	10 oz	12 oz

MAIN MEAL No. 8

(Recipes 11, 18, 23)

FOOD	PORTIONS PER CALORIE TOTAL		
	600	750	1050
Fruit cocktail	1 c	1½ c	2 c
Top round beef	4 oz	5 oz	8 oz
Egg noodles	½ c	½ c	1 c
Carrots and onions (cooked)	½ c	1 c	1 c
Green pepper, stuffed	¼	½	
Whole grain bread, cornbread, or bran muffin	1 sl	1 sl	2 sl
butter	1 t	1 t	2 t
Skim milk	8 oz	10 oz	12 oz

MAIN MEAL No. 9

(Recipes 1–7, 11, 25)

FOOD	PORTIONS PER CALORIE TOTAL		
	600	750	1050
Salad	1½ c	1½ c	1½ c
dressing			
Baked ham	4 oz	5 oz	9 oz
Pineapple ring or sweet potato	1	2	3
Peas, black-eye	⅓ c	½ c	1 c
Whole grain bread or muffin	1 sl	1 sl	2 sl
butter	1 t	1 t	2 t
Skim milk	8 oz	10 oz	12 oz

MAIN MEAL No. 10

(Recipes 1–7, 14, 19)

FOOD	PORTIONS PER CALORIE TOTAL		
	600	750	1050
Lettuce leaves	3	4	4
dressing	1 T	1 T	1 T
T-bone steak	4 oz	5 oz	8 oz
Potatoes, boiled	2	3	3
Carrots, cooked	½ c	½ c	1 c
Tomato	1 sl	2 sl	2 sl
Whole wheat bread	1 sl	1 sl	2 sl
butter	1 t	1 t	2 t
Skim milk	8 oz	10 oz	12 oz

MAIN MEAL No. 11

(Recipes 1–7, 22, 26)

FOOD	PORTIONS PER CALORIE TOTAL		
	600	750	1050
Salad	1½ c	1½ c	1½ c
dressing	1 T	1 T	1 T
Hamburger, broiled	4 oz	4–5 oz	8 oz
Potato, baked (or potato salad)	½	1	1
Lima beans in tomato sauce	½ c	½ c	1 c
Carrot sticks or tomato slices	3	4	5
Whole grain bread or bran muffin	1 sl	1 sl	2 sl
butter	1 t	1 t	2 t
Skim milk	8 oz	10 oz	12 oz

MAIN MEAL No. 12

(Recipes 10, 27, 28)

FOOD	PORTIONS PER CALORIE TOTAL		
	600	750	1050
Okra (or tossed salad)	1½ c	1½ c	1½ c
Baked veal loin chop	4 oz	5 oz	8 oz
Rice, cooked	½ c	¾ c	1 c
Stewed or baked tomatoes	½ c	½ c	1 c
Whole wheat bread	1 sl	1 sl	2 sl
butter	1 t	1 t	2 t
Skim milk	8 oz	10 oz	12 oz

MAIN MEAL No. 13

(Recipes 1–7, 11, 16, 23, 58)

FOOD	PORTIONS PER CALORIE TOTAL		
	600	750	1050
Salad	1½ c	1½ c	1½ c
dressing	1 T	1 T	1 T
Roast beef, top round	4 oz	4–5 oz	8 oz
Baked potato	½	1	1
butter	1 t	1 t	1 t
Zucchini or green and gold squash	1 c	1 c	1 c
Whole wheat bread or muffin	1 sl	1 sl	2 sl
butter	1 t	1 5	2 t
Skim milk	8 oz	10 oz	12 oz

MAIN MEAL No. 14

(Recipes 1–8, 30)

FOOD	PORTIONS PER CALORIE TOTAL		
	600	750	1050
Salad	1½ c	1½ c	1½ c
dressing	1 T	1 T	1 T
Trout, bluefish, or perch fillet	5 oz	6 oz	9 oz
Potato, mashed	½ c	1 c	1 c
butter	1 t	1 t	1 t
Broccoli with tart sauce	½ c	½ c	1 c
Beets, cooked	½ c	½ c	1 c
Whole grain bread	1 sl	1 sl	2 sl
butter	1 t	1 t	2 t
Skim milk	8 oz	10 oz	12 oz

MAIN MEAL No. 15

(Recipes 19, 31)

FOOD	PORTIONS PER CALORIE TOTAL		
	600	750	1050
Celery and carrot sticks	2 (1 ea)	2	4
Steak, bottom round	4 oz	4–5 oz	8–9 oz
Potatoes, broiled	2	2	3
Brussels sprouts casserole	1 srv	1 srv	1 srv
Whole grain bread	1 sl	1 sl	2 sl
butter	1 t	1 t	2 t
Skim milk	8 oz	10 oz	12 oz

MAIN MEAL No. 16

(Recipes 1–7, 32)

FOOD	PORTIONS PER CALORIE TOTAL		
	600	750	1050
Tossed salad	1½ c	1½ c	1½ c
dressing	1 T	1 T	1 T
Breaded fish, fish sticks or fish patties with lemon wedge	4 oz	4–5 oz	8 oz
Corn on the cob (5″ x 1¾″)	1	1	2
Whole grain bread	1 sl	1 sl	2 sl
butter	1 t	1 t	2 t
Skim milk	8 oz	10 oz	12 oz

MAIN MEAL No. 17

(Recipes 1–7, 33, 34 or 14)

FOOD	PORTIONS PER CALORIE TOTAL		
	600	750	1050
Salad	1½ c	1½ c	1½ c
dressing	1 T	1 T	1 T
Meat loaf	4 oz	4 oz	8 oz
Potato, scalloped	½ c	1 c	1 c
Peas, green	½ c	½ c	1 c
Whole grain bread	1 sl	1 sl	2 sl
butter	1 t	1 t	2 t
Skim milk	8 oz	10 oz	12 oz

MAIN MEAL No. 18

(Recipes 35, 36)

FOOD	PORTIONS PER CALORIE TOTAL		
	600	750	1050
Coleslaw with mayonnaise	1 c	1 c	1 c
Fried chicken	4 oz	6 oz	8 oz
Corn on the cob (5″ by 1¾″)	1	1	2
Biscuit	2	3	3–4
butter	1 t	2 t	3 t
Skim milk	8 oz	10 oz	12 oz

MAIN MEAL No. 19

FOOD	PORTIONS PER CALORIE TOTAL		
	600	750	1050
Greens	1 c	1 c	1 c
oil and vinegar	1 T	1 T	1 T
Baked rib veal chop	4 oz	4–5 oz	8 oz
Corn	½ c	¾ c	1 c
Onion	¼ c	¼ c	½ c
Whole wheat bread	1 sl	1 sl	1 sl
butter	1 t	1 t	1 t
Skim milk	8 oz	10 oz	12 oz

MAIN MEAL No. 20

FOOD	PORTIONS PER CALORIE TOTAL		
	600	750	1050
Tossed salad	1½ c	1½ c	1½ c
dressing	1 T	1 T	1 T
Spaghetti, meatballs, romano cheese and tomato sauce	1 c	1½ c	2 c
Extra meatballs	1 oz	1 oz	2 oz
Italian or garlic bread	1 sl	1 sl	2 sl
butter	1 t	1 t	2 t
Skim milk	8 oz	10 oz	12 oz

MAIN MEAL No. 21

(Recipes 1–7, 37)

FOOD	PORTIONS PER CALORIE TOTAL		
	600	750	1050
Tossed salad	1½ c	1½ c	1½ c
dressing	1 T	1 T	1 T
Beef loaf, carrot coins	1 srv	1 srv	1½ srv
Potato, mashed	½ c	¾ c	1 c
Whole grain bread	1 sl	1 sl	2 sl
butter	1 t	1 t	2 t
Skim milk	8 oz	10 oz	12 oz

MAIN MEAL No. 22

(Recipes 1–7, 38, 39)

FOOD	PORTIONS PER CALORIE TOTAL		
	600	750	1050
Salad	1½ c	1½ c	1½ c
dressing	1 T	1 T	1 T
Swiss steak	4 oz	4 oz	8 oz
Green beans, Peking	½ c	1 c	1 c
Whole wheat bread	1 sl	1 sl	2 sl
butter	1 t	1 t	2 t
Skim milk	8 oz	10 oz	12 oz

MAIN MEAL No. 23

(Recipes 1–7, 40, 41)

FOOD	PORTIONS PER CALORIE TOTAL		
	600	750	1050
Salad	1½ c	1½ c	1½ c
dressing	1 T	1 T	1 T
Liver loaf	1 srv	1 srv	1½ srv
Spanish snap beans	½ c	1 c	1 c
Whole wheat bread	1 sl	1 sl	2 sl
butter	1 t	1 t	2 t
Skim milk	8 oz	10 oz	12 oz

MAIN MEAL No. 24

(Recipes 1–7, 42, 43)

FOOD	PORTIONS PER CALORIE TOTAL		
	600	750	1050
Salad	1½ c	1½ c	1½ c
dressing	1 T	1 T	1 T
Stuffed fish	4 oz	5 oz	8–9 oz
Peanut stuffed peppers	1	1	1½
Whole wheat bread	1 sl	1 sl	2 sl
butter	1 t	1 t	2 t
Skim milk	8 oz	10 oz	12 oz

MAIN MEAL No. 25

(Recipes 1–7, 44, 45)

FOOD	PORTIONS PER CALORIE TOTAL		
	600	750	1050
Salad	1½ c	1½ c	1½ c
dressing	1 T	1 T	1 T
Salmon loaf	1 srv	1 srv	1½ srv
Stuffed celery	1 srv	2 srv	3 srv
Whole wheat bread	1 sl	1 sl	2 sl
butter	1 t	1 t	2 t
Skim milk	8 oz	10 oz	12 oz

MAIN MEAL No. 26

(Recipes 1–7, 46, 48)

FOOD	PORTIONS PER CALORIE TOTAL		
	600	750	1050
Salad	1½ c	1½ c	1½ c
dressing	1 T	1 T	1 T
Fish à la stroganoff	1½ srv	2 srv	4 srv
Squash, baked	½ c	½ c	1 c
Whole grain bread	1 sl	1 sl	2 sl
butter	1 t	1 t	2 t
Skim milk	8 oz	10 oz	12 oz

MAIN MEAL No. 27

(Recipes 1–7, 49, 50)

FOOD	PORTIONS PER CALORIE TOTAL		
	600	750	1050
Salad	1½ c	1½ c	1½ c
dressing	1 T	1 T	1 T
Flounder Kiev	1 srv	1 srv	2 srv
Hot slaw	1 srv	1 srv	1 srv
Whole grain bread	1 sl	1 sl	2 sl
butter	1 t	1 t	2 t
Skim milk	8 oz	10 oz	12 oz

MAIN MEAL No. 28

(Recipes 1–7, 51)

FOOD	PORTIONS PER CALORIE TOTAL		
	600	750	1050
Salad	1½ c	1½ c	1½ c
dressing	1 T	1 T	1 T
Braised beef slimmer	1 srv	1 srv	1½ srv
Whole grain bread	1 sl	1 sl	2 sl
butter	1 t	1 t	2 t
Skim milk	8 oz	10 oz	12 oz

MAIN MEAL No. 29

(Recipes 1–7, 52)

FOOD	PORTIONS PER CALORIE TOTAL		
	600	750	1050
Salad	1½ c	1½ c	1½ c
dressing	1 T	1 T	1 T
Chinese pepper steak	1 srv	1 srv	1½ srv
Bean sprouts	½ c	¾ c	1 c
Whole wheat bread	1 sl	1 sl	2 sl
butter	1 t	1 t	2 t
Skim milk	8 oz	10 oz	12 oz

MAIN MEAL No. 30

(Recipes 1–7, 53)

FOOD	PORTIONS PER CALORIE TOTAL		
	600	750	1050
Salad	1½ c	1½ c	1½ c
dressing	1 T	1 T	1 T
Lasagna	1 srv	1 srv	1½ srv
Whole wheat bread	1 sl	1 sl	2 sl
butter	1 t	1 t	2 t
Skim milk	8 oz	10 oz	12 oz

MAIN MEAL No. 31

(Recipes 1–7, 54–56)

FOOD	PORTIONS PER CALORIE TOTAL		
	600	750	1050
Salad	1½ c	1½ c	1½ c
dressing	1 T	1 T	1 T
Hi-Pro tofu casserole	1 srv	1 srv	1½ srv
Green beans, stir fry	½ c	¾ c	1 c
Zucchini skillet medley	1 srv	1 srv	1 srv
Potatoes au gratin	½ c	½ c	1 c
Whole grain bread	1 sl	1 sl	2 sl
butter	1 t	1 t	2 t
Skim milk	8 oz	10 oz	12 oz

MAIN MEAL No. 32

(Recipes 1–7, 57, 58)

FOOD	PORTIONS PER CALORIE TOTAL		
	600	750	1050
Salad	1½ c	1½ c	1½ c
dressing	1 T	1 T	1 T
Carrot tofu	1 srv	1 srv	1½ srv
Celery oriental	1 srv	1 srv	1 srv
Brown rice	½ c	½ c	1 c
Bean sprouts	½ c	½ c	½ c
Whole grain bread	1 sl	1 sl	2 sl
butter	1 t	1 t	2 t
Skim milk	8 oz	10 oz	12 oz

MAIN MEAL No. 33

(Recipes 1–7, 11, 14 or 30, 59)

FOOD	PORTIONS PER CALORIE TOTAL		
	600	750	1050
Salad	1½ c	1½ c	1½ c
dressing	1 T	1 T	1 T
Eggaroni	1 srv	1 srv	1½ srv
Broccoli	½ c	½ c	1 c
Muffin	1	1	2
butter	1 t	1 t	2 t

MAIN MEAL No. 34

FOOD	PORTIONS PER CALORIE TOTAL		
	600	750	1050
Salad	1½ c	1½ c	1½ c
dressing	1 T	1 T	1 T
Pizza	1 sl	1 sl	2 sl
Carrot sticks	2	3	4
Skim milk	8 oz	10 oz	12 oz

Recipe Index

Beans	14, 26, 39, 41, 56
Beef	19, 23, 33, 37, 38, 51, 52, 53
Biscuits, muffin, cornbread	11, 18, 36
Fish	8, 32, 42, 44, 46, 49
Ham	25
Lamb	9
Liver	17, 40
Macaroni	60
Potatoes	14, 16, 22, 34
Poultry	12, 21, 35
Rice	10
Salads	1–7 (22)

Note: The recipes given here have been developed in the food research laboratories of the Institute of Home Economics in the Department of Agriculture unless otherwise noted.

Recipes No. 1–7

Salads

1. Lettuce, carrot, green pepper, radish
2. Grated carrots, diced celery, cucumber slices
3. Spinach, endive or lettuce, with tomato wedges
4. Sliced raw cauliflower flowerets, lettuce, chopped green pepper, celery, pimento
5. Shredded cheese, cucumber cubes, celery slivers
6. Cooked red kidney beans, thinly sliced celery, sweet onions
7. Cooked cut green beans, crisp bacon bits, sweet pickles, onion rings

Recipe No. 8

Broiled Fish (4 servings)

1 lb. fish fillets
salt and pepper
3 to 4 tablespoons melted butter or oil

Preheat broiler. Cut fillets into serving pieces. Sprinkle with salt and pepper.

Grease broiler rack lightly. Place fish on rack, skin side up. Brush with melted butter or oil.

Place rack 2 to 3 inches from heat. Broil fish 5 to 8 minutes or until brown. Baste with butter or oil. Turn, baste other side, and broil until brown.

Recipe No. 9

Pan-broiled Lamb Chops

Loin, rib, or shoulder chops may be used. Heat a heavy frying pan very hot and grease lightly. Lay chops in pan and brown quickly on both sides. Turn thick chops on side. Reduce heat and cook slowly, turning often. Do not add water and do not cover. From time to time, pour off excess fat.

Note: Chops ¾ to 1-inch thick take 10 to 15 minutes to cook.

Recipe No. 10

Oven-cooked Rice

2 cups boiling water
½ teaspoon salt
1 cup rice

Measure boiling water into a baking dish and add salt. Stir in the rice.

Cover and bake at 350°F about 35 minutes.

Recipe No. 11

Bran Muffins (12 muffins)

2 c sifted whole-wheat flour
3 T bran
2 t baking powder
½ t salt
1 T sugar
1 egg, beaten
1 c milk
¼ c melted shortening or oil

Sift together whole-wheat flour, bran, baking powder, salt, and sugar.

Combine egg, milk, and shortening. Add to the dry ingredients all at once, stirring only enough to moisten.

Fill greased muffin pans two-thirds full. Bake at 400°F about 20 minutes.

Recipe No. 12

Roast Turkey

Sprinkle inside of turkey with salt. Stuff body and neck cavities loosely. Brush skin of turkey with melted butter.

Place turkey breast side up on rack in shallow pan. Cover turkey loosely with aluminum foil. Do not cover pan; do not add water.

Salt the giblets, seal in aluminum foil and roast along with the turkey. Or, simmer them in salted water until tender.

Cook at 325°F. Baste turkey several times with drippings or melted butter.

The turkey is done when the leg joints move easily and the flesh on the leg feels soft and pliable when pressed with the fingers.

Roasting times:

WEIGHT (LBS)	TIME AT 325°F FOR STUFFED CHILLED TURKEY
4–8	3 –4½ hrs.
6–12	3½–5 hrs.
12–16	5 –6 hrs.
16–20	6 –7½ hrs.
20–24	7½–9 hrs.

Recipe No. 13

Bread Stuffing

This recipe is for 1 quart of ½-inch crumbs torn from sliced bread. The guide below indicates how many quarts you will need for the size of turkey to be roasted. Multiply each ingredient in this recipe by the number of quarts needed.

⅓ c butter
¾ c chopped celery
3 T chopped parsley
2 t chopped onion
1 qt bread crumbs
½ t savory seasoning
½ t salt
pepper to taste

Melt the butter in frying pan, add celery, parsley, and onion and cook a few minutes. Add to crumbs with the seasoning. Mix lightly but well.

TURKEY WEIGHT (LBS)	QUARTS OF BREAD CRUMBS NEEDED
4–8	1–2
6–12	2–3
12–16	3–4
16–20	4–5
20–24	5–6

Recipe No. 14

Creamed or Scalloped Vegetables

(asparagus, lima beans, snap beans, broccoli, cabbage, carrots, cauliflower, celery, onions, peas, potatoes, spinach)

For four servings, use 2 cups cooked vegetable and 1 cup thin or medium white sauce (see Recipe No. 15).

To cream, simply mix vegetables with white sauce and heat thoroughly. Potatoes and lima beans, because they are drier than other vegetables, may be best with the thin sauce.

To scallop cooked vegetables, combine them with white sauce in a baking dish and top with bread or cracker crumbs mixed with melted butter. Bake at 350°F until the mixture is heated through and the crumbs are browned.

Recipe No. 15

White Sauce (for creamed and scalloped vegetables, gravy, etc.)

Thin	*Medium*
1 c milk	1 c milk
1 T flour	2 T flour
1 T butter (or cooking fat or oil)	1–2 T butter (or cooking fat or oil)

Melt butter (or fat) and blend in the flour to make a smooth mixture. Add milk slowly and cook over very low heat, stirring constantly until thickened. Add salt to taste (about 1/4 teaspoon for each cup of milk used). Cook 3 to 5 minutes longer, stirring occasionally.

Recipe No. 16

Stuffed Baked Potaotes or Sweet Potatoes

Bake medium potatoes or sweet potatoes at 425°F until soft (about 35 to 60 minutes).

Cut slice off top of potato, scoop out inside. Mash potato and season with salt and butter. Add pepper and hot milk to white potatoes, cinnamon to sweet potatoes.

Stuff shells with the mashed potato and put back in oven a few minutes to brown.

Recipe No. 17

Broiled Liver

Place 1/3" liver cut into serving sizes on broiling rack, 3 inches from the heat source. Brush with melted butter. Broil one minute on each side. Garnish with onion, lemon, or parsley.

Recipe No. 18

Cornbread (6 servings)

1/3 c sifted flour
3/4 c yellow cornmeal
1 1/2 t baking powder
1 t sugar
1/2 t salt
1 egg, beaten
2/3 c milk
2 T melted shortening or oil

Sift together the flour, cornmeal, baking powder, sugar and salt.

Combine the egg, milk, and shortening or oil. Add to dry ingredients and stir only enough to mix.

Pour batter into a greased 8″ by 8″ baking pan. Bake at 425°F 25 minutes.

Recipe No. 19

Broiled Steak

Choose a steak 1 to 2 inches thick, trim fat. Preheat broiler. Grease broiler rack lightly. Place steak on rack so that the top of meat is 2 to 3 inches below source of heat—3 inches if the steak is to be cooked well-done.

Broil the steak until top side is well browned, season, then turn and brown the other side.

STEAK THICKNESS	BROILING TIME (minutes)
1 inch	
rare	about 10
medium	about 15
well-done	20–25
1½ inches	
rare	about 15
medium	about 20
well-done	25–30
2 inches	
rare	about 25
medium	about 35
well-done	45–50

Recipe No. 20

Beets in Orange Sauce (6 servings, 1/2 cup each)

3 c drained sliced beets, canned or cooked
1 T butter
2 T lemon juice
3/4 c orange juice
2 T cornstarch
3/4 t salt
1/8 c sugar

Mix cornstarch, salt and sugar in a saucepan. Stir in the orange juice and cook until thickened, stirring constantly. Remove from heat and stir in lemon juice and butter. Pour sauce over beets and heat.

Recipe No. 21

Roasted Chicken

Follow recipe No. 12 for roasted turkey. A 2½ to 4½ pound roaster will require ½ to 1¼ quarts of stuffing and will take 2 to 3½ hours to roast.

Recipe No. 22

Potato Salad (6 servings)

(Courtesy American Egg Board)

4 cups cubed, warm, cooked and peeled potatoes (4–6 medium)
1/4 c bottled Italian dressing
1 c mayonnaise or salad dressing
1 c chopped celery
1/2 c finely chopped green pepper
1/4 c finely chopped onion
1 t salt
5 hard-cooked eggs, coarsely chopped
1 hard-cooked egg, sliced

Pour Italian dressing over potatoes while warm; let stand while preparing remaining ingredients. Stir in mayonnaise, celery, green pepper, onion, and salt. Gently stir in chopped eggs. Cover; chill for several hours to blend flavors. Garnish with sliced egg.

Recipe No. 23

Roast Beef

Rub the meat with salt, pepper, and flour, and brown on all sides in a little melted butter or oil in a deep heavy pan.

Slip a low rack under meat to keep it from sticking to pan. Add 1/2 cup water; cover pan closely.

Cook slowly over low heat until done—about 3 hours. Add more water as needed.

During the last hour, cook vegetables with meat.

Make gravy with the liquid.

Recipe No. 24

Stuffed Green Peppers (4 servings)

4 medium green peppers
1/4 c chopped celery
1 c cooked rice
1/4 c chili sauce
1/2 c grated cheese
1/4 t salt
2 T butter
Bread or cracker crumbs

Cut out stem ends of peppers and remove seeds. Boil peppers 5 minutes in salted water; drain.

Melt butter and cook celery in it until tender.

Mix all ingredients.

Fill peppers with rice mixture; top with crumbs. Place in a half-inch of hot water in a baking dish.

Bake at 350°F until peppers are tender and crumbs browned (about 30 minutes).

Recipe No. 25

Baked Ham (4 servings)

1 lb. slice of ham
1 sliced pineapple (or 2 medium peeled sweet potatoes)
1 T brown sugar or honey
1 c hot water

Cut ham in serving pieces and brown lightly in a fry pan.

Place the ham in a baking dish. Place pineapple or sweet potato slices over it, and lightly sprinkle with sugar.

Add water to drippings, pour over ham. Cover. Bake at 350°F about 45 minutes, basting occasionally with the liquid. Remove cover to brown for the last 15 minutes.

Recipe No. 26

Lima Beans in Tomato Sauce (4 servings)

1 c dry lima beans
3 c water
¾ t salt
½ c chopped onion
1 c cooked or canned tomatoes

Boil beans in the water for 2 minutes. Remove from heat and let soak one hour or overnight if more convenient.

Add ½ t salt to the beans and boil gently 45 minutes. Drain. Add tomatoes and rest of the salt.

Boil gently until beans are tender—about 30 minutes, stirring occasionally to keep from sticking. Add a little more water or tomato if the mixture gets too dry.

Recipe No. 27

Panned Vegetables

(cabbage, kale, collards, spinach, okra, summer squash, or zucchini)

Finely shred cabbage, kale, collards, or spinach. Slice okra, summer squash, or zucchini thin.

For 4 servings use 2 quarts spinach, 1 quart cabbage, kale or collards; 3 cups okra or summer squash. Measure vegetable after cutting.

Heat 2 tablespoons butter in a heavy frying pan. Add vegetables and sprinkle with salt. Cover pan to hold in steam. Cook over low heat; stir once in a while.

Cabbage will be done in 5 to 10 minutes; other vegetables take longer.

Recipe No. 28

Baked Tomatoes

Wash medium-sized tomatoes, ripe or green, and cut off the stem ends. Place tomatoes in a baking dish. Sprinkle tops with salt and pepper and bread or cracker crumbs mixed with butter. Add just enough water to cover bottom of dish.

Cover and bake at 375°F until tomatoes are soft (about 30 minutes for ripe tomatoes, 45 minutes for green tomatoes).

When tomatoes are about half done, uncover the dish to brown the crumbs.

Recipe No. 29

Green and Gold Squash

(Courtesy of Mollie Stein)

3/4 lb. medium zucchini
3/4 lb. yellow squash
1 medium onion chopped

- 2 T salad oil
- 2 T chopped parsley
- ½ t salt
- ½ t oregano
- ½ t pepper
- 3 eggs, slightly beaten
- ½ c milk
- 1 c shredded sharp cheddar cheese
- ½ c crushed saltine cracker crumbs

Scrub squash and zucchini well, cut off stem ends. Shred coarsely. Sauté onion in oil in large frying pan until golden brown. Remove from heat. Stir in squash, zucchini, parsley, oregano, salt, pepper, and slightly beaten eggs blended with milk. Spoon one-half mixture into greased 1½ quart casserole. Sprinkle with half of the cheese and cracker crumbs. Make a second layer with rest and top with rest of cheese and crumbs. Bake at 325°F for 45 minutes.

Recipe No. 30

Broccoli with Tart Sauce (4 servings)

- 1 bunch broccoli (about 1 pound)
- ½ t salt
- ½ t sugar or honey
- ½ t paprika
- 2 T lemon juice
- 2 T butter
- 1½ t prepared horseradish

Trim off tough outer layer of large broccoli stalks and split the stalks. Cook in lightly salted boiling water about 10 minutes. Drain.

Blend salt, sugar, and paprika. Add lemon juice, butter, and horseradish. Mix well and pour over the broccoli.

Recipe No. 31

Brussels Sprouts Casserole (4 servings)

1½ T butter
½ c chopped celery
¼ c chopped onion
1½ T flour
½ t salt
pepper
1 c tomatoes
1½ c cooked brussels sprouts
Fine bread or cracker crumbs mixed with melted butter

Heat the butter in a fry pan. Add the celery and onion and cook slowly until they are yellow.

Blend in the flour, salt, and pepper, and add the tomatoes. Stir and cook until the mixture is thick.

Put the brussels sprouts into a greased baking dish and add the tomato mixture. Sprinkle the crumbs over the top.

Bake at 350°F about 30 minutes.

Recipe No. 32

Fish Patties (4 servings)

1½ c flaked cooked or canned fish
1½ c mashed potatoes
1 T finely chopped onion
½ t salt
1 egg
pepper
flour
butter or oil

Combine all ingredients except flour and butter or oil. Shape mixture into patties, roll in flour and brown in butter or oil.

Recipe No. 33

Meat Loaf (4–5 servings)

1 lb. ground beef or veal
1/4 lb. sausage or salt pork
1/4 c chopped onion
1/8 c chopped celery
1/8 c chopped parsley
1/2 c soft bread crumbs
1/2 c milk or canned tomatoes
1 egg, beaten
1/2 t salt
pepper

Mix all ingredients together thoroughly. If salt pork is used, cut it into small pieces and fry until lightly browned before adding to the other ingredients.

Mold mixture into a loaf. Place on tough paper or foil on rack in uncovered pan.

Bake at 350°F for 1½ to 2 hours. Serve hot or cold.

Recipe No. 34

Scalloped Potatoes (4 servings)

3 medium potatoes, pared and sliced
1 T flour
1 t salt
pepper
1 c hot milk
1 T butter

Put a layer of potatoes in a greased baking dish and sprinkle with some of the flour, salt, and pepper. Repeat until all the potatoes are used. Pour milk over potatoes and dot with butter.

Cover and bake at 350°F for 30 minutes. Remove cover and continue baking until potatoes are tender (about 30 minutes). If potatoes are not brown enough on top, place the uncovered dish under the broiler for 3 to 5 minutes.

Recipe No. 35

Fried Chicken

1½–3 lbs. chicken
salt, pepper, flour
oil

Cut chicken into serving pieces. Season with salt and pepper and roll in flour.

Heat oil (about ½-inch deep) in a heavy frying pan. Put the thickest pieces of chicken in the oil first. Do not crowd. Cook slowly, turning often. Do not cover pan. The thickest pieces will take from 20 to 35 minutes to cook.

After the pieces have been browned, cooking may be finished in a moderate (350° F) oven if desired.

French-fried chicken

Dip chicken in thin batter made with 1 cup sifted flour, 1 egg, ¾ cup milk, and ½ teaspoon salt. Heat in a deep pan to 365°F. Fry 10 to 15 minutes.

Recipe No. 36

Biscuits (8 2-inch biscuits)

1 c sifted flour
1 t baking powder
⅜ t salt
⅙ c shortening
⅜ c milk

Sift flour, baking powder and salt together. Cut or rub in shortening until well blended.

Slowly mix in milk, using just enough to make dough that is soft but not sticky.

Turn dough onto a lightly floured board and knead a few strokes. Roll or pat to ¾-inch thickness. Cut with a biscuit cutter or cut into squares.

Place on a baking sheet and bake at 450°F about 15 minutes.

Recipe No. 37

Carrot Coins Beef Loaf (10 servings of 1 slice each)

2 lbs. ground beef (80 percent lean)
5 long carrots
1 can (16 oz) tomatoes
1¾ t salt
1⅛ t leaf oregano
¼ t pepper
½ c crushed crackers
2 medium onions, cut in ¼″ slices
1 egg
1 small green pepper, cut in thin strips
1 c sliced celery
½ c water
1 T cornstarch

Cook carrots (whole) in boiling water in large covered frying pan 15 minutes; drain. Drain tomatoes, reserving juice; cut tomatoes into large pieces. Stir ¾ cup of reserved tomato juice, 1½ teaspoons salt, 1 teaspoon oregano and pepper into cracker crumbs in large bowl. Chop enough onion slices to make ¼ cup. Add ground beef, chopped onion and egg to cracker-crumb mixture; mix lightly but thoroughly. Place ⅓ of mixture in 9″ x 5″ loaf pan, pressing into layer in bottom of pan. Place 2 carrots lengthwise in pan and press into meat mixture. Top with layer of second ⅓ of meat mixture. Place 1 carrot down the center and press into meat. Add remaining meat mixture to form layer and press last 2 carrots into top, covering them with meat. Bake in a moderate oven (350°F) for 1 hour 15 minutes or until done.

For vegetable sauce, add remaining onion slices, green pepper, celery, ¼ teaspoon salt and ⅛ teaspoon oregano to boiling water in saucepan. Cover tightly and cook 15 minutes or until vegetables are almost tender. Combine cornstarch with remaining reserved tomato juice and pieces of tomatoes. Gradually combine with vegetables and cook 3 to 5 minutes, stirring until thickened. Slice meat loaf in 10 equal slices and serve with vegetable sauce.

Receipe No. 38

Swiss Steak (4 servings)

1 lb. beef or veal rump or round, cut about 1-inch thick
salt and pepper
flour
butter or oil
2 c cooked or canned tomatoes or tomato juice

Season meat with salt and pepper, sprinkle with flour. Pounding helps make the meat tender. Cut meat into serving pieces and brown in a little butter.

Add tomatoes or juice, cover, and simmer gently until meat is tender (about 1½ hours).

Recipe No. 39

Green Beans Peking

(Courtesy of Mollie Stein)

3 T butter
1 t soy sauce
1 chicken bouillion cube
1 (16 oz) can whole green beans
dash ground ginger, celery salt, white pepper

Melt butter, add rest of ingredients and blend. Cover and heat beans through.

Recipe No. 40

Liver Loaf (8 servings)

1½ lbs. liver
2 T butter or oil
¼ c chopped onion
¼ c chopped celery
¼ lb pork sausage

- 1 t salt
- 1 c bread crumbs
- 1 egg, beaten
- 2/3 c milk or canned tomatoes

Brown the liver lightly in the butter. Chop fine.

Brown the onion and celery in the butter and add to the liver. Add the rest of the ingredients, using just enough milk or tomatoes to moisten the mixture well.

Pack firmly into a loaf pan. Bake at 350°F 1½ to 2 hours.

Recipe No. 41

Spanish Snap Beans (4 servings)

- 1 T butter
- 1 T chopped onion
- 1/3 c chopped green pepper
- 1 c tomatoes
- 1½ c cooked snap beans
- salt and pepper
- toasted bread crumbs

Heat the butter and brown the onion and green pepper in it. Add tomatoes and cook slowly about 15 minutes.

Add beans and season to taste with salt and pepper. Heat thoroughly. Turn into serving dish and top with bread crumbs.

Recipe No. 42

Baked Stuffed Fish (6 to 8 servings)

- 3 lbs. dressed fish
- 1½ t salt
- 1 quart bread stuffing (See Recipe No. 13)
- 4 T melted butter or oil

Wash and dry the fish. Sprinkle inside and out with salt. Fill body cavity of fish loosely with stuffing. Close with skewers or sew opening with needle and cord.

Place fish in greased pan; brush with butter (1 strip of bacon can be laid over top, if desired). Bake at 350°F 40 to 60 minutes.

Recipe No. 43

Peanut-Stuffed Peppers (4 servings)

4 green peppers
1 T melted butter
1/3 c uncooked rice
3 T finely chopped onion
1/4 c chopped celery
1 t salt
1 c water
1 1/3 c cooked or canned tomatoes
2/3 c chopped salted peanuts
1/4 c fine bread or cracker crumbs mixed with 1 T melted butter

Cut out stem ends of the peppers and take out the seeds. Cook peppers 5 minutes in boiling salted water.

Combine the butter, rice, onion, celery, and salt in a frying pan.

Add water slowly as the mixture begins to cook and simmer covered 5 to 10 minutes. Add tomatoes and simmer 10 minutes longer or until rice is almost done, adding more liquid if needed, stir in peanuts.

Stuff peppers with the mixture and sprinkle with crumbs. Place peppers in a baking dish with a little hot water and bake at 350°F 30 to 40 minutes.

Recipe No. 44

Salmon Loaf (4 servings)

2 c flaked canned or cooked salmon
3 T butter or oil
3 T flour
1 c milk and salmon liquid
salt and pepper
2 T finely chopped parsley
2 c bread crumbs
1 egg, beaten
(1 t grated onion, optional)

Drain canned salmon, saving the liquid.

Make sauce: Heat butter, blend in flour. Add enough milk to the salmon liquid to make 1 cup, and stir in the flour mixture. Cook until thickened, stirring constantly. Season.

Mix the sauce with the other ingredients. Form into loaf. Bake in uncovered pan at 350°F about 30 minutes or until brown. (1 teaspoon grated onion can be added to mixture before baking for extra flavor.)

Recipe No. 45

Stuffed Celery (6 servings)

½ t Worcestershire sauce
½ c cottage cheese
⅓ c (about 2 each, 2″ by ⅝″) chopped sweet gherkins
¼ t salt
1 T chopped celery leaves
6 celery stalks, cut in 8-inch pieces

Combine Worcestershire sauce, cottage cheese, gherkins, salt and celery leaves; mix well. Spread cheese mixture on celery stalks.

Recipe No. 46

Fish à la Stroganoff (6 servings)

6 frozen raw breaded fish portions ($2\frac{1}{2}$ or 3 ounces each)
2 T butter, melted
paprika
2 c cooked egg noodles
2 T butter
1 t poppy seeds
Stroganoff sauce (see Recipe No. 47)
Chopped parsley

Place frozen fish portions in a single layer on a well-greased baking pan, 15″ by 10″ by 1″.

Pour melted butter over portions. Sprinkle with paprika.

Bake at 500°F for 15 to 20 minutes or until brown and fish flakes easily when tested with a fork.

Combine noodles, butter, and poppy seeds. Arrange noodles on a warm serving platter and place fish portions on top. Pour the stroganoff sauce over the portions. Sprinkle with parsley.

Recipe No. 47

Stroganoff Sauce (2–$2\frac{2}{3}$ cups)

1 4 oz.-can, drained sliced mushrooms
½ c chopped onion
1 clove garlic, finely chopped
2 T butter, melted
1 $10\frac{1}{2}$ oz-can of condensed cream of chicken soup
¼ t paprika
¼ t salt
dash pepper
1 c sour cream

Cook mushrooms, onion, and garlic in butter until tender. Add soup and seasonings. Cook over low heat for about 10 minutes, stirring occasionally. Add sour cream. Heat.

Recipe No. 48

Baked Squash

Cut acorn squash in half, Hubbard squash in 3 to 4-inch squares. Remove seeds. Place squash in baking pan.

Sprinkle squash with salt and dot with butter. Pour a little water into the pan. Cover.

Bake at 400°F until squash is partly done (about 30 minutes for acorn, 45 minutes for Hubbard).

Uncover and continue baking until squash is soft (about 20 minutes for acorn, 30 for Hubbard).

Recipe No. 49

Flounder Kiev (6 servings)

2 lbs. flounder fillets
½ c butter, softened
2 T chopped parsley
1 T lemon juice
¾ t Worcestershire sauce
¼ t liquid hot pepper sauce
1 clove garlic, finely chopped
½ t salt
dash pepper
2 eggs, beaten
2 T water
½ c flour
3 c bread crumbs
butter for frying

Combine butter, parsley, lemon juice, Worcestershire sauce, liquid hot pepper sauce, and garlic. Place mixture on waxed paper and form into a roll. Chill sauce until firmly set.

Skin fillets. Cut fillets into 12 strips, about 6 x 2 inches. Sprinkle fish with salt and pepper.

Cut sauce roll into 12 pieces. Place a piece at one end of each strip of fish. Roll fish around sauce and secure with a toothpick.

Combine egg and water.

Roll fish into flour. Dip fish in egg and roll in crumbs. Chill for 1 hour.

Fry in deep butter or fat at 350°F for 3 to 5 minutes or until brown and fish flakes easily when tested with a fork.

Drain on absorbent paper. Remove the toothpicks.

Recipe No. 50

Hot Slaw (4 servings)

- 2 eggs
- 1/4 c water
- 3 T vinegar
- 1/2 t salt
- 1/4 t powdered dry mustard
- a few celery seeds
- 1 T butter
- 1 pint finely shredded cabbage

Beat the eggs, add the water, vinegar, salt, mustard and celery seeds.

Cook, stirring frequently, until thick. Add the butter.

Stir in the cabbage, and mix thoroughly with the dressing. Cover and heat a few minutes.

Recipe No. 51

Braised Beef Slimmer (4 servings)

(Courtesy of National Livestock and Meat Board)

- 1 1/2 lbs beef bottom round steak, cut 3/4-to-1-inch thick
- 1 t salt
- 1/2 t thyme
- 1/8 t pepper
- 1 beef bouillion cube
- 1/2 c hot water
- 2 packages (10 ounces each) cut Italian green beans, defrosted

8 oz mushrooms, sliced
3/4 cup buttermilk
1 T cornstarch

Trim separable fat from steak; slowly heat fat in large frying pan or Dutch oven to obtain 1 tablespoon drippings. Discard fat. Cut steak into 3/4–1-inch cubes; brown in drippings. Pour off drippings. Combine salt, thyme, and pepper and sprinkle over meat. Crush bouillion cube and dissolve in hot water; add to meat, cover tightly, and cook slowly 1 1/2 hours. Stir in green beans and mushrooms; continue cooking, covered, 13 minutes. Add buttermilk to cornstarch, stirring to blend; gradually add to meat mixture and cook until thickened, stirring occasionally. Continue cooking 2 minutes.

Recipe No. 52

Chinese Pepper Steak (4 servings)

(Courtesy of National Livestock and Meat Board)

1 1/4 lbs top round steak, cut 3/4 to 1-inch thick*
1 T cornstarch
1/2 t sugar
1/4 t ginger
1/4 cup soy sauce
3 medium green peppers
3 small tomatoes
2 T cooking oil
1 clove garlic, minced
1/4 cup water

Partially freeze steak to firm and slice diagonally across the grain into very thin strips. Combine cornstarch, sugar and ginger and stir in soy sauce. Pour mixture over meat and stir. Cut green peppers into thin strips and cut tomatoes into wedges. Quickly brown beef strips (1/3 at a time) in hot oil and

*1 flank steak (approximately 1 1/4 pounds) can be used

remove from pan. Reduce heat; add green pepper, garlic and water to pan and cook until green pepper is tender-crisp 5 to 6 minutes. Stir in meat and tomatoes and heat through.

Recipe No. 53

Lasagna (8 servings)

- 1/2 lb. ground beef
- 4 ozs lasagna noodles
- 2 T butter
- 1/2 c finely chopped onion
- 1 finely chopped garlic clove
- 1 6-oz can tomato paste
- 1 20-oz can tomatoes
- 1 t salt
- 1/8 t pepper
- 1/4 t basil
- 1/4 t oregano
- 1/2 pound ricotta or cottage cheese
- 1/2 pound Swiss cheese slices
- 1/4 c Parmesan cheese, grated

Cook lasagna noodles until tender, following package directions. Drain.

Separate lasagna and hang over edge of colander or pan to allow for easy handling later.

While lasagna is cooking, melt butter in large frying pan. Add onion and garlic and cook over moderate heat until tender. Add ground beef, and cook slowly, stirring frequently until red color disappears from meat.

Stir in tomato paste, tomatoes, salt, pepper, basil, and oregano. Simmer 30 minutes, stirring occasionally.

In an 8-inch square baking dish, make three layers of meat sauce, lasagna, and ricotta, Swiss, and Parmesan cheeses. Use about 1/3 of each for each layer, topping with Parmesan cheese.

Bake at 350°F until mixture is bubbly and cheese is lightly browned (about 35 to 40 minutes). Cut into 8 portions.

Recipe No. 54

Hi-Pro Tofu Casserole (4 servings)

(Courtesy of Pat Raisher)

12 ozs tofu
1 t salt
1 c milk
½ cup bread crumbs
2 oz skim mozarella cheese (grated)
4 t oil
2 T butter
2 onions (thinly sliced)
1 c cooked brown rice

Preheat oven to 350°F. Heat skillet and coat with oil and butter. Add onion and sauté till browned. Add rice, then tofu, and cook 2 minutes longer. Season with salt. Place mixture in casserole that has been oiled. Pour in milk, then sprinkle with bread crumbs and cheese. Bake 20 minutes until browned.

Recipe No. 55

Zucchini Skillet Medley (6 servings)

(Courtesy of Mollie Stein)

¼ c safflower oil
¾ c sliced celery
½ c sliced onion
1 clove garlic, minced
1 lb unpeeled zucchini, sliced ¼-inch thick (about 4 cups)
2 tomatoes, cut in eighths
½ cup green pepper strips
½ cup shredded peeled carrots
1 8 oz can tomato sauce
2 t prepared yellow mustard
¼ t dried basil leaves
¾ t salt
⅛ t pepper

Heat oil in 12″ skillet over medium heat. Add celery, onion, and garlic; sauté until tender. Add zucchini, tomatoes, green pepper and carrot. Sauté 10 minutes.

Stir in remaining ingredients. Reduce heat and simmer 5 minutes or until vegetables are tender, stirring occasionally. Serve hot or cold.

Recipe No. 56

Stir-Fry Green Beans (6 servings)

(Courtesy of Mollie Stein)

- 1½ lbs. fresh green beans
- 3 T butter
- 1½ t salt
- ¼ t pepper
- ⅛ t leaf dried marjoram

Wash and cut beans diagonally in 1-inch pieces. Melt butter in skillet. Add beans and sprinkle with salt and pepper and marjoram. Cover and cook 5 minutes over medium high heat. Uncover and cook 3 minutes longer, stirring constantly.

Recipe No. 57

Carrot Tofu Burgers (Serves 8)

(Courtesy of Pat Raisher)

- 30 oz tofu
- 6 T grated carrots
- 4 T minced onion
- 2 T sunflower seeds (ground)
- ¾ t salt
- oil for sautéing

Cut tofu in slices and squeeze out all moisture. Combine with carrots, onions, seeds and salt in large bowl. Mix well and knead as if kneading bread. When mixture is smooth and holds together, moisten palms with warm water and shape into 8 patties. Sauté in oil until brown on both sides. Drain briefly, then serve topped with low-salt soy sauce.

Recipe No. 58

Celery Oriental

6 to 8 large outside celery stalks, sliced diagonally
1 c sliced fresh or canned mushrooms
1/4 c toasted almond halves

Cook celery in a little boiling water until crisply done. Drain. Sauté mushrooms in 3 T butter. Add celery and almonds. Toss lightly until heated.

Recipe No. 59

Eggaroni (6 servings)

(Courtesy American Egg Board)

2 T butter
2 T flour
2 c milk
6 hard-cooked eggs, sliced
2 c cooked elbow macaroni (approx. 1/2 of 7-oz pkg)
1/2 c chopped celery
2 T finely chopped onion
1 1/2 t oregano, crushed
1 t salt
1/8 t pepper
3 T grated Parmesan cheese
Tomato wedges
Parsley, optional

Melt butter in 10-inch skillet; blend in flour. Cook, stirring until mixture is smooth and bubbly. Stir in milk all at once; heat to boiling, stirring constantly. Boil and stir until mixture is smooth and thickened. Reserve 4 center egg slices for garnish; chop remaining eggs. Stir chopped eggs, macaroni, celery, onion, oregano, salt and pepper into white sauce. Pour into greased 2-quart casserole. Sprinkle Parmesan cheese over top of casserole. Bake in preheated 350°F oven 25–30 minutes. Garnish with tomato wedges, reserved egg slices and parsley, if desired.

11

Vitamin and mineral supplements are an important part of any reducing diet. Even the Food and Drug Administration, not noted for encouraging the public to take vitamin supplements, recognizes the need for supplements when dieting.

The Slendernow Diet emphasizes good nutrition, not just minimal nutrition, for optimal nutrition is required to protect the body against the extra stresses of dieting.

It is extremely difficult for a diet with fewer than 2400 calories to provide the recommended allowance of the B-complex vitamins, iron and calcium. These are usually lacking even in fat-producing diets.

The U.S. Health and Nutrition Examination Survey (HANES) of 1971–1972 found that diets of nearly 50 percent of the American people contained less than the daily recommended levels in one or more essential vitamins and minerals.

For example, only 80 percent of the diets provided the Recommended Dietary Allowance (RDA) for protein, 28 percent provided the RDA for vitamin A, 39 percent provided the RDA for calcium, 48 percent provided the RDA for vitamin C, and 64 percent provided the RDA for iron.

The most serious problem, however, is not this restriction of the nutrient intake due to reduced food quantity, but the effects of mental and physical stresses during dieting that rob your bodies of the nutrients that you do manage to eat.

Just the act of resisting a delicious snack is a mental stress. When you become hungry because your blood-sugar level drops, that is a physical stress.

Mental and physical stresses can be gauged by the types and amounts of the various hormones that are released in the body during stress and accumulate in the urine. It has been found that some diets cause considerably more stress than others, but all reducing diets can cause some stress.

One common sign of stress is irritability. It is often said that the first thing lost during a diet is your temper. Severe diets also lead to fatigue, depression, sleeplessness and other symptoms of stress. These effects can be alleviated with proper nutrition.

Stress due to dieting not only produces undesirable symptoms, it slows the burning of body fat. The body uses vitamins and minerals to manufacture the hormones produced during stress, thus they are unavailable to convert body fat to energy.

Even if you did manage to get nearly the recommended daily allowance of the B-complex vitamins, they are quickly consumed during the stress of dieting. Therefore, your needs have increased, and frequent replenishment by vitamin and mineral supplementation is the most sensible way of meeting your increased needs.

During stress, the small amount of vitamin C stored in the adrenal cortex is consumed or spilled into the blood. Thus vitamin C stores are depleted easily during stress, and unless the stores are replenished, the body is not fully protected.

Deficiency Slows Fat Loss

If you don't supply your body with what it needs, your body will crave more food in a subconscious effort to get more nutrients. But craving for more food is *not* what is needed during dieting. You will still lose weight if you are deficient in vitamins and minerals; but more of that weight loss will be from muscle or other lean (protein) tissue.

As already noted, a person can convert only a given amount of fat into energy in a day, due to the limited supply of the necessary fat-mobilizing enzymes. When you cut back your intake of calories so severely that your body cannot make up the calorie deficit with the conversion of the fat it can mobilize into energy, then the body must burn lean tissue.

There's another limit to the fat-burning process. When there is less than optimal amounts of the B-complex vitamins and certain minerals, the body doesn't produce as many of the fat-burning enzymes. Thus more lean tissue is consumed as fuel for life-sustaining energy. The idea of dieting is to lose fat—not the vital lean tissue that holds your figure and provides strength.

An additional bonus of proper vitamin and mineral supplementation during dieting is that, provided you also drink plenty of fluids, you will prevent constipation due to reduced food bulk, a very common complaint of dieters. The B-complex vitamins are especially critical to regularity.

Table 11.1 lists the suggested vitamins and minerals that should be included in any reducing diet. It is best to take the suggested quantities in two doses to better replenish the water-soluble B-complex vitamins and vitamin C.

TABLE 11.1

Suggested vitamin and mineral supplement (these are *minimum* levels)

NUTRIENT	MINIMUM LEVEL
Vitamin A	10,000 i.u.
Vitamin D	50 i.u.
Vitamin E	50 i.u.
Vitamin C	250 mg
Folic Acid	200 mcg
Vitamin B-1	20 mg
Vitamin B-2	20 mg
Niacinamide	20 mg
Vitamin B-6	20 mg
Vitamin B-12	20 mcg
Biotin	10 mcg
Pantothenic Acid	20 mg
Bioflavonoids	25 mg
Choline	20 mg
Inositol	20 mg
PABA	20 mg

The following minerals should also be supplied

Potassium	Magnesium
Calcium	Copper
Iodine	Zinc
Iron	Manganese

Fiber

Adding bran to the Diet Shakes occasionally helps to maintain regularity. Bran can also be mixed into foods at the main meal or taken as chewable tablets. Complex carbohydrates are an essential part of the main meal, but extra complex carbohydrates can be added any time regularity becomes a problem. Carrots, celery, lettuce, cabbage and other fibrous vegetables can be added to the meal or eaten as snacks.

Water

Water is not usually considered a supplement, but you need "extra" water to maintain regularity. Food largely consists of water, even though we think of it as dry. The water is incorporated into the cells of plants and animals. Dehydrated foods are foods with most of the water removed. They occupy only a fraction of the space that they would if the water were there. When the quantity of food is reduced during dieting, the water intake is also reduced. The reduction in bulk and water combine to cause irregularity.

The Slendernow Diet purposely includes full glasses of water at midmorning and midafternoon. It is important that you remember to drink them.

Laxative

No laxative is required on the Slendernow Diet. The complex carbohydrates, water, B-Complex vitamins and mild exercise all help keep regularity. However, should you find yourself concerned about regularity, keep the following two natural laxatives in mind.

Lax-A-Shake

Add three tablespoons of whole bran to any of the Diet Shake recipes (omit ice).

Prune Shake

Juice Mix (omit ice)
4–6 oz prune juice
2 tablespoons whole bran

12

The *secret* reason behind your weight gain over the past few years is not that you are eating more food but that your metabolism has slowed because you are not as active. Children are a bundle of motion and burn more calories for energy. On the other hand, adults become less active each year. They participate in fewer sports, accumulate laborsaving devices, have the children run more errands for them, and sit still longer. All of these put a brake on the metabolism rate.

Knowing this, you are still probably tinkering with the idea of passing up this chapter. You may not feel that exercise is really that important to dieting. You may not enjoy exercising. You may feel that you don't have the time. You are too far out of shape. You know all there is to know about exercising and will be bored reading this chapter. Excuses go on and on.

It's your life. You're the one who wants to lose weight and look better. If you decide not to exercise, you have actually made the decision that you will accelerate your decline into poor shape and poor health. You can only maintain your status quo by exercising enough to maintain your present level of conditioning.

Don't forget that those who exercise feel better than those who don't.

There are some new developments that make exercise more enjoyable, more effective, less boring, and less time-consuming.

According to the National Center for Health Statistics, Americans on the average were 4 pounds heavier in 1974 than they were a decade earlier, even though they consumed fewer calories. The weight gain is a fat gain, not due to slightly increased height, and not due to muscle gain. The reason for becoming fatter on fewer calories is caused mostly by a more sedentary lifestyle. Other factors include food quality and meal timing, both of which increase insulin level in the blood and result in more blood sugar being converted to fat.

The *NIH Record*, a publication of the National Institutes of Health, commented on the studies that indicate that lack of physical activity is more often the cause of overweight than overeating.

> These studies—comparing the food intake and activity patterns of obese persons with those of normal weight—showed that the obese people did not consume more calories but that they were less active.
>
> The idea that increased physical activity increases appetite is untrue. A lean person in good health may eat more following increased activity, but the extra exercise burns up the extra calories.
>
> Adding 30 minutes per day of moderate exercise to your schedule can result in a loss of up to 25 pounds in 1 year, assuming the food intake is the same. (*NIH Record*, p. 3, February 22, 1979)

We must return to a more active lifestyle or at least exercise regularly. If you are active, you do not need to exercise because you are using your body all day. If you are inactive, you don't use your body much, so remember the adage about your body: Use it—or lose it.

INCREASED METABOLISM

One reason that many people don't bother to exercise is that they read where you have to run a zillion miles or exercise 24 hours a day to burn off a few pounds. Such articles are misleading because they discuss the number of calories required to move the muscles to do the work for that activity. They ignore the more important fact that regular exercising causes the body to change its metabolic gears.

One of the main reasons that most people put on flab is not that they eat more but that they exercise less. The "double-barreled blast" of expending fewer calories in activity and slowing metabolism, while still eating the same amount of food, can cause obesity. Many former athletes can attest to this. Stronger muscles burn more fat all day long, even when you're resting or sleeping. Consistent exercise increases the amount of the fat-burning enzymes in the muscles.

The increase in basal metabolism that occurs with regular exercise has been verified by scientific tests by several sports medicine researchers, such as Dr. Dave Costill of Ball State University (Congress on Sports Medicine, Washington, D.C., May 1978).

> While most people think of exercise as a means to use calories and thereby reduce many people don't realize that your body composition may make a difference too. A fat 150-pound person will use fewer calories sitting still than a lean, muscular 150-pound person. Fat tissue simply doesn't use many calories. It is essentially inert from that point of view. Muscle fibers use calories even when you are at rest. Developing and maintaining good strong muscles will help prevent obesity. (*The Health Letter,* June 27, 1980)

Exercise must be regular and last a sufficient length of time in order for the body to change metabolic gears and shake up its energy-producing mechanism by burning fat.

Regular moderate exercise requires your body to maintain an improved state of readiness to convert fat to energy. If you make only rare demands for sustained energy production, the body conserves enzymes and energy by shutting down this fat-to-energy mechanism.

The best way to help burn excess fat through exercise is with a pleasant, moderate exercise program that is convenient, family oriented, safe, and economical. Sounds great, but does it exist? Swimming is certainly good exercise but not always convenient, and for those living in cold wintertime temperatures, the expense of joining an indoor pool can be prohibitive. Jogging seems to be the fad of the day—if it's your thing by all means do it. Unfortunately, Dad's pace is a little faster than Mom's or the kids so if it's an exercise for the entire family you're looking for, jogging may not be the best choice. However, as I'll discuss shortly, there are several pleasant and effective exercises from which to choose.

OTHER BENEFITS

Proper exericse will speed up your fat-burning rate at the same time it firms your figure, but there are more benefits as well. Exercise stimulates muscle repair, improves circulation, tones and stimulates your internal organs, chases the blues, eases stress, improves immunity, improves sex, improves sleep, lowers blood cholesterol, helps you think better, strengthens bones, and leaves you with a good feeling and alertness for 10 to 12 hours afterwards.

Data from the American Cancer Society shows that men over 45 who exercise regularly have a death rate 4 times lower than those who don't. Dr. Paul Metzer, Associate Medical Director for Nationwide Insurance Co. says, "Just because you are past 40, don't think you are too old for regular exercise. Ten minutes of exercise will double the blood level of norepinephrine, a hormone related to adrenalin, which boosts your spirits and destroys depression."

Dr. Gabe Mirkin, who teaches Sports Medicine at the University of Maryland, says that a 15-minute walk can be more soothing than the most popular tranquilizers on the market today.

Exercise increases your ability to withstand pain by increasing your production of the body's pain-killing compound beta-endorphin, according to the *New England Journal of Medicine* (560, September 3, 1981).

It is now widely accepted that moderate exercise is a preventative against heart disease. An interesting review of the effect of exercise on heart health has been published in *The New England Journal of Medicine* (302, 18: 1026–1027, May 1, 1980) by Drs. Ralph Paffenbarger and Robert Hyde.

In the article, Paffenbarger and Hyde review how exercise increases maximal oxygen uptake, slows the heart, normalizes blood pressure, decreases ventricular ectopic activity, increases the myocardial capillary-to-fiber ratio, enlarges the bore of the coronary arteries, increases cardiac output, increases physical work capacity, lowers total blood cholesterol, lowers triglycerides, lowers low-density lipoprotein (a bad guy), and increases high-density lipoprotein (a good guy).

The article goes on to show that the evidence is clear that

physical inactivity is far more detrimental to health than any hazards of strenuous exertion. Other studies have shown that exercise can cut the heart death rate in half.

IS A CHECKUP NEEDED?

It used to be stressed that anyone should have a physical examination before starting an exercise program, especially if he was over 40 years old. It has been estimated that millions of people were scared away from exercise by this advice. Some never started exercising because of fear, others because of the time and expense required for the physical examination and exercise-stress test.

Now that advice is changing in an effort to encourage more people to exercise. After all, using your body wisely is not a condition requiring medical blessings—unless you are ill or refuse to exercise properly.

Drs. P. Astrand and K. Rodhal summed it up in their *Textbook of Work Physiology* (McGraw-Hill, 1970): "Anyone should submit to a thorough medical checkup before deciding *not* to exercise."

The National Heart, Lung and Blood Institute now says flatly that most people up to 60 do not have to see a doctor before they start exercising, "since a gradual, sensible exercise program will have minimal health risk." Their new pamphlet, "Exercise and Your Heart," concludes that not exercising regularly is far more dangerous than refraining because of an unwillingness to see a doctor first.

Well, that's dandy if you feel fine and have no symptoms and are under 60, but for others—and to be doubly sure yourself—simply ask your doctor when you consult with him about going on a diet if you need a checkup before exercising.

Slendernow Exercise Program

The Slendernow Diet Exercise Program is designed to increase fat burning, improve your figure and strength and keep you from getting bored. The exercises are rhythmic, aerobic, and increase cardiovascular fitness.

You will begin gradually and build up your conditioning so that you can exercise for 10–12 minutes, four days a week. There are several suggested metabolism-increasing exercises to choose from. The suggested plan would be a brisk walk on Monday evening, rebounding on Tuesday evening, no exercise on Wednesday, a brisk walk on Thursday, and rebounding on Friday. The weekend is free for whatever activities you can find to enjoy.

You can add figure-shaping exercises as you please, and you can adjust the 4-day-a-week exercise plan to your own preference. Of course, you can exercise longer if you desire. It seems that most people can always squeeze in ten minutes of exercise, but they put off doing a half hour, and, as a result, they do no exercises.

The Slendernow Diet Exercise Program does not encourage "all-out" exercise. Such strenuous activity can lead to injury and exhaustion while burning comparatively little body fat. Dr. David Costell has found that at maximum effort, the body can burn essentially nothing but carbohydrate fuel, so that at the maximal rates of energy burning, the body does not burn fat because it is inefficient for it to do so.

A runner keeping a five-minute-mile pace is deriving 90 to 100 percent of his energy from carbohydrate, while a runner going slower at *half* that speed can derive 50 to 60 percent of his energy from body fat.

The secret to the most efficient fat-burning exercise is to loosen up by mild stretching and bending for a few minutes, then walk slowly, then walk or exercise briskly (but not near your maximum speed) for ten to fifteen minutes. More if you please.

Now let's look at some excellent exercises for burning body fat.

STRIDING

The best all-around fat-burning exercise is striding—that is, walking briskly at the pace of a military march, or 120, 30-inch steps per minute. This pace is easily achieved by humming or whistling a march (any will do, but to activate your memory, consider John Philip Sousa's march, "Stars and Stripes Forever").

Striding is less strenuous on the feet and knees than jogging, but more importantly, it allows a family or group of friends to stay together and even talk as they exercise. If you prefer to jog, of course, then go ahead and jog. But do so because you enjoy it, not because you think it's better for burning calories. It is not.

Yes, the energy charts show that jogging burns more calories per minute than striding, but you finish a distance course sooner by jogging. The total energy burned is a function of the calories burned per minute times the duration of the exercise. Regardless of the speed that you travel, you will burn approximately the same number of *calories per mile.* This figure depends on many factors (including how high you lift your feet, how much you swing your arms, how much weight you are carrying, and your present metabolic efficiency) but typically amounts to between 90 and 120 *calories per mile.* It is a law of physics that if you move the same weight the same distance, you do the same amount of work. Speed or duration has nothing to do with it. Thus, you will burn up 3,500 extra calories—which is the equivalent of one pound of body fat—whenever you stride or jog an extra 35 miles. Remember, it makes no difference which—stride or run—and it makes no difference if you do it in a day, a week, a month, or a year. Cover an extra 35 miles, keep all other activity the same, and you will weigh one pound less than you would otherwise.

Now remember the bonus: if you exercise regularly and moderately, you step up your metabolism and burn fat—even while you are showering and sleeping.

One study showed that regular walking alone can account for a decent weight loss over a year. Walking 30 minutes daily amounted to an average loss of 22 pounds in a group of overweight women.

Striding is a healthy habit that you can follow all the years of your life and you can begin at any age in almost any condition. You can even stop to smell the roses as you improve your circulation and nourish your cells.

Striding is moderate exercise so there is no oxygen debt. If tightness, pressure, or pain in the chest ever occurs, you can stop and immediately reestablish normal conditions.

You don't have to stride each exercise period. You can switch exercises to prevent boredom.

On bad-weather days, you can switch with the next night's exercise or substitute a completely different exercise. As an example, I recommend regular exercise alternating between striding and rebounding. On rainy or snowy nights, I prefer to substitute stair climbing, high kicking, or rope jumping in place of striding.

REBOUNDING

Rebounding is growing in popularity because it is effective, fun, and can be done indoors even while watching TV. Rebounding is running or jumping in place on a trampolinelike device that absorbs the shock and stress that jogging can place on the skeletal system. Rebounders are "mini-trampolines" about 40 inches in diameter and are easily portable so that they may be used in any room or office. They are widely available. If you don't have one, you could use a bed or couch.

Executives are finding that rebounding helps them relieve stress as well as improve their heart rate. Women like the soft feeling as they jog or bounce and they feel no strain on their backs.

Start your rebounding by gradually bouncing on the rebounder. As you begin to bounce a little higher, extend your arms out to the sides at shoulder height and make circular loops. Small loops help the muscles in the back, neck, and shoulders. Large loops make the exercise similar to jumping rope.

After loosening up for a minute or so, jog in place, gradually bringing your knees and feet higher. Continue for awhile but not until the point of exhausting your muscles. If you are in good shape, you can sprint in place for a few seconds.

Next, shuffle your feet back and forth as you bounce. This will rest some of your muscles while maintaining aerobic conditions (proper pulse and breathing) to produce cardiovascular efficiency.

After an interval of shuffling, jog in place, only this time lift your heels up to nearly touch your buttocks. Again, do not exhaust your muscles.

Next, as you bounce, cross your legs and feet as you twist your trunk in the opposite direction. Reverse the twist on alternative bounces. This helps firm the waistline, hips, and stomach.

Continue to alternate the exercises. At first, you may not be able to rebound much longer than a minute. If this is the case, rebound as long as you can without exhausting yourself. Rest until your pulse returns to normal and then repeat. Continue to alternate exercise and rest until you have exercised for a total of ten minutes.

An alternative would be to rebound for a while and then stride or climb stairs to make up the full 10-minute exercise period.

It won't be long until you are rebounding for more than ten minutes without resting. You can dance and have a good time as you melt away the pounds.

JUMPING ROPE

An alternative to either striding or rebounding is jumping rope.

Go into any sports store and you will be shown cotton ropes with wood handles, nylon ropes with ball bearings in the handles, leather ropes with weights in the handles, and variations thereof, including models with digital counters in the handles so that you don't have to count as you jump. Any of them are fine—so is the simple clothesline.

A rope is portable, compact, and lends itself to progressive exercising. If jumping rope isn't fun, then why do fun-loving young girls spend hours at it? Don't worry, you won't have to spend too much time to get a good workout for your heart and lungs. Ten to twelve minutes will be sufficient.

HIGH KICKS

One of my favorite bad weather alternatives is the "high kick." High kicks are both aerobic and tummy flattening. Rheo

Blair (nutritionist to the stars) taught me a particularly effective form of high kicks.

Here is how Rheo suggests doing them:

> Rise on the toes, then while keeping each leg straight—locked at the knee—KICK your right foot as high as you can, bring it down, and KICK your left foot as high as you can, alternating with each leg, and keep doing this until you are moderately tired.
>
> In the beginning, 10 repetitions, which is 5 kicks with each leg, is probably enough for one set. Then, after you have rested a bit, you can do another set of 10 repetitions, which is 5 kicks with each leg. Rest a few minutes more, or you can even wait, and do another set of 10 repetitions—5 kicks with each leg—just before you go to bed. As you become more conditioned, and as you become more flexible, you will find that you will be able to do more repetitions during each set.
>
> Please take it easy at first! Remember, some of those muscles have not been used for years—and they will cry out to high heaven, poor things!
>
> When you are able to do a hundred perfect high kicks, which is 50 repetitions with each leg, you will be in much better condition than you are now. You will also notice that the exercise stimulates proper breathing, and will definitely increase your endurance and lung power. You will find this an enjoyable exercise; it is most delightful. You will also find, after taking a warm bath or a shower, that it is much easier to kick even higher, as your muscles will be more supple.

STAIR CLIMBING

Another exercise is stair climbing. Climb 250 steps, or walk up and down your stairs for ten to twelve minutes. Don't run or push yourself. Just cover the distance in a comfortable manner. You can burn an extra 4 calories for every 10 steps climbed, but more importantly you are stepping up your metabolism by regular, moderate exercise.

TUMMY FLATTENERS

The above exercises are the backbone of the Slendernow Diet program, but you may wish to add a few "tummy flatteners" to help shape you as you lose inches from your waist.

A trim, flat look is a sign of youth. As people age and become more sedentary, the abdominal muscles lose strength and collapse outward. Fat accumulates in the membranes holding the intestines together and presses the abdominal muscles out farther. You can lose the fat, but still have the sagging belly. So, let's shape up!

There are four main muscles in the abdominal wall that we want to strengthen to produce that youthful look. The rectus abdominus muscles are long, flat muscles that form the front of the abdomen. Most people think these muscles are one muscle that covers the belly, but they are two, one lining each side of the front abdomen. The rectus abdominus are crossed by fibrous bands called tendinous inscriptions.

There are also three big sheets of muscle along the back and sides of the abdomen that lie atop each other in layers. The outermost layer is made up of the external obliques. The fibers in this layer run diagonally. The middle layer is made up of the internal obliques, which have fibers running diagonally in the opposite direction. The innermost layer is the transversus abdominus, which has fibers that run horizontally.

The external obliques help bend the spinal column sideways and rotate the spinal column in one direction. The internal obliques also help bend the spinal column, but they rotate the spinal column in the opposite direction. The transversus abdominus is the prime constrictor muscle of the abdomen. *This muscle alone holds the secret of making the abdomen compact* and giving a "V" shape to your trunk.

The following exercise is the most effective for strengthening the tummy-flattening transversus abdominus, and it is not a sit-up or leg-raise!

Stand erect, take a shallow breath (not a big one) and hold it. Now slowly start to draw your entire abdominal wall inward. Keep pulling your abdomen in, harder and harder. Imagine that you are trying to make your front abdominal wall touch your spinal column. Hold it in very hard for a full ten seconds and then relax. Rest a moment and then repeat once. In a few weeks, this will give you a flat, slightly convex abdomen that accents your chest.

This brief anatomy lesson points out why different exercises are required to strengthen and firm the entire abdomen. Some people like to also firm the rectus abdominus because it is the abdominal covering that can be touched. The popular sit-up and leg-raise variations do firm the rectus abdominus somewhat but are really not that good for slimness.

Dr. Ellington Darden, exercise expert and author of *Weight Loss, Body Shaping and Slenderizing,* comments, "The belief that sit-ups and leg-raises are abdominal exercises is a misconception. These movements work the hip flexors and only mildly involve the abdominals."

Drs. Alan Halpern and Eugene Bleck analyzed five sit-up positions and came away with a new exercise that should revolutionize the strengthening of the abdomen. Five sit-up positions are identified as A, B, C, D, and E.

A. The classic, or traditional, sit-up position of lying on one's back, legs flat and feet together, where the hands are extended during the sit-up to touch the toes corresponding to the hands.

B. The same positioning as A, only opposite hands touch opposite feet, alternately one side at a time.

C. Bent-knee sit-up, hands behind head with no twisting in the trunk during the sit-up.

D. Same bent-knee sit-up as C with twisting of the trunk while sitting up to touch elbow—first right, then left—to opposite knee.

E. Same bent-knee sit-up as in C and D except that the individual raises himself only enough to elevate the scapula from the mat.

In terms of the percentages of muscular activity occurring during the respective sit-up cycles (A–E), the values are given in Table 12.1.

You can see that the best variation is the "E" variation involving the shoulder lift. You can choose your favorite, if you do decide to do sit-ups, at least ten every day are essential. You can do more if you desire, but do at least the minimum.

TABLE 12.1

SIT-UP VARIATION	PERCENT OF MUSCULAR ACTIVITY RECTUS ABDOMINUS	EXTERNAL OBLIQUE (AVERAGE OF RIGHT AND LEFT)
A	34	22.5
B	37	20
C	48	35
D	48+	35+
E	93	90

(Source: Clinical Orthopedics Vol. 145, pp. 172–178, 1979.)

IF YOU CAN'T DO SIT-UPS

What can you do if you can't do sit-ups of any variation? You can strengthen yourself to the point that you can.

A reverse sit-up can be done to prepare you for doing sit-ups. Sit on the floor with your knees bent. Place your heels near your buttocks with your feet flat on the floor. Place your hands to the sides and slightly to the rear for support. Tuck your chin against your chest. Curve your back, ease up on your arms, and gently lower your back to the floor as you "uncoil."

Repeat this exercise 10–20 times daily for a week.

Now you are ready for a sit-down. Sit on the floor, but this time place your feet forward and spread several inches apart. Spread your knees apart. Straighten your back. Grasp your outer thighs at midthigh and bend your elbows up and out. Lower your back until the small of your back touches the floor.

Now, let go of your legs and place your arms over your head. Hold this position for 8 to 10 seconds. It is important that the small of your back remains on the floor. If it doesn't, start the exercise holding onto your thighs a little higher and putting a rounded curve in your back.

Repeat this exercise ten times daily for a week.

After a week, try doing a sit-up. If you can't, continue the above program until you can. Once you can do a sit-up, you will soon be able to do two, then three, and so on.

You have to add a little exercise to your life to reap its benefits. You'll be glad you did. Maybe other lifestyle changes would be good for you too.

13

Lifestyle Adjustment For Permanent Control

You soon will reach your targeted weight. But what will happen after?

If you decide that you are going to revert back to your former habits that made you overweight, my response is simply that your health belongs to you! You may choose habits of life or habits of death. It is your choice and it is your responsibility.

Your lifestyle is the single most important factor in maintaining your desired weight for more than a year. In *Psychosomatic Medicine* (37:195, 1975), Dr. A. J. Stunkard reviewed 30 different studies where the superiority of behavioral modification (lifestyle adjustment) was demonstrated over other methods of weight maintenance after weight reduction.

Behavior modification is a scientific name for learning a few tricks. At first, many of the suggestions seem trivial, but they really do make a big difference over the course of a lifetime.

Keep in mind that just 200 extra calories a day can add 20 pounds of fat a year. That's only 17 potato chips or a small biscuit with butter and jelly. Four extra pieces of fudge (500 calories) daily would put 50 pounds of fat a year on you.

Weight gain is usually a slow process that creeps up on you. If you detect and eliminate the "little" habits that cause the gain, you can forget about dieting. So, pay attention to the "little" suggestions and see how many you can incorporate into your lifestyle. This chapter will not only make those suggestions, it will help you implement them.

Actually, you are not going to give up any pleasure; you are merely going to substitute a healthier pleasure than overeating to reward yourself. Most of us are taught that sweets are rewards. You will learn better treats than extra calories, and you will learn more constructive ways to beat boredom or depression.

You will learn that sometimes you eat snacks just because you receive a "cue" to eat. Many "cues" come from our environment and friends. These cues can be removed or ignored once they are understood. Cues can be avoided or blocked by understanding how they work and their effect on you, and then by planning ahead.

It is natural to ask yourself why you overeat when you know it makes you fatter and unhappier. It takes strong willpower to resist the reward of the pleasing taste, smell, and sight of food when it is placed before you, when the punishment occurs much later as you stand on the scale. Your best chance is to prevent the reward from coming before you. This is achieved by design.

Numerous studies have shown that eating is environmentally controlled and that no amount of threat can overcome bad habits cued by environmental factors (time of day, passing the refrigerator, meeting with friends, and so on).

Keeping detailed records of where and when you eat will help you identify eating cues, and thus help you change them. Cues are often reduced by such tactics as eating in one room only and doing nothing else while eating.

Imagery training is a useful aid. You can use positive daydreams rather than food to provide comfort or reward during stress. Also you can daydream about the "new you" that you are building to help you reject bad habits.

I am a nutritionist, not a behavioral psychologist. Therefore, I consulted with a pioneer in using behavioral modification in weight control to design the behavioral modification portion of the Slendernow Diet Program.

The Slendernow Neighborhood Clubs of America assisted in finding the optimal program, choosing from several behavioral modification programs that have already been developed. Excellent results were obtained using the program created at the University of Arkansas by Drs. Rick Guyton and Jerry Lafferty. Their complete program is described in their book, *Breaking the Eating Habit* (available from Health Habits,

2870 Crossover Rd., Fayetteville, Arkansas, 72701). I highly recommend it.

Dr. Guyton has graciously permitted me to add major aspects of his program to the Slendernow Diet Program.

Remember that the Slendernow Diet Program is an eight-week program. It is also a course in improving your lifestyle. During the program, it is essential that continuous records be kept.

This will help identify the types of behavior that need to be reinforced and the ones which need to be modified. The idea of the Slendernow Diet Program is that reeducation and modification of personal habits are the most effective and only permanent way to maintain your desired weight.

Let's look at a few suggestions to help you reduce and maintain your desired weight.

MEAL TIPS

Place utensils down and place hands in lap while chewing food. Take small bites and chew food at least 15 times before swallowing.

Use smaller plates (salad plates instead of dinner plates) and more shallow bowls at all main meals. Always leave a little on the plate.

Fill your plate in the kitchen and don't go back for seconds. Do not place bowls or platters of food on your dining table. If you are dining alone, prepare enough for only one serving of each food item at each meal. (This saves money, time, and waste.)

Eat all meals at a designated eating place, preferably the kitchen or dining room table. Do not read or watch television while eating. (Your food is more satisfying if you pay attention to it, and if you're distracted, you may lose track of how much you've eaten.)

Take time to enjoy your meals. The slower you eat, the better your appetite control keeps up with the amount of food consumed. If you gulp food, you will overshoot and eat more than your body needs to turn off hunger.

Arrive at the table a few minutes after everybody else has begun eating, but stop when they stop. Never be the last one to leave the table or make others wait for you to finish. When serving, serve yourself last—there will be less to tempt you.

Introduce a two-to-five-minute conversation break halfway through the meal. Converse without eating. Then resume a slower, relaxed meal.

Become a connoisseur of food; concern yourself with quality, not quantity.

Maintain daily records of your eating behavior utilizing the forms in this chapter. By being conscious of what you eat and why you eat, you'll eat less.

Don't be afraid to say, "No, thank you." It's your body, your health, and your life. No one else has the right to force food on you.

Keep a thermos of ice water or weak iced tea on your desk for use when spontaneous "coffee breaks" occur. This is in addition to your midmorning and midafternoon glass of water.

Set the bread platter away from you at restaurants and at home. If you must linger over coffee, clear the table or ask the waiter to clear the table.

Take your vitamin supplements in divided doses to replenish the water-soluble B-complex vitamins and vitamin C. Take one portion with your breakfast Diet Shake and a second portion before the main meal. Taking a vitamin with water before the main meal helps to fill you up.

Know the approximate calorie value of foods and choose the lower calorie alternative if you have a choice. A baked potato is better than potatoes au gratin or french fries.

Never go to a party feeling hungry (they won't have many nutritious low-calorie foods there) or tired (you'll yield to temptation). Eat your main meal before you go, but perhaps leave out 100–200 calories. When food is served, treat yourself once and don't go back.

You *can* go back to non-calorie food—carrots, celery, and so forth—but stay away from the dips and salted items.

March to the side of the room opposite from the food. Keep busy conversing. If you feel that you need a drink in your hand, ask for a diet drink with lemon twist. Use plenty of ice.

SHOPPING, STORAGE, AND PREPARATION TIPS

Remove all snack foods from the house. If others demand snacks, have them store the snacks in a special area that you are not exposed to. Try to talk them into avoiding ready-to-eat snacks—if a snack has to be prepared, it is less likely to be eaten. Ask your family to give you needed support.

Remove all food items usually in view on counters to new areas out of sight.

Store refrigerated foods in opaque containers.

Plan your weekly menus in advance and shop once a week for the main meal items. Perishable items should be bought at least 24 hours ahead of time. Shop only from a prepared list and never buy on impulse. Shop only on a full stomach and prepare the list on a full stomach. Shop alone.

If you are eating out, plan your meal in advance when you are not hungry. While there, converse, dance and keep busy before and after the meal.

Substitute fresh or water-packed fruits for syrup-packed fruits, and plain frozen vegetables for those in butter sauce. Remove skin and loose fat from chicken. Cut away all visible fat from meats. Soften butter before using so that it spreads better and you use less. Use spice for flavoring, and less salt.

Substitute tomato juice for tomato sauce; skim milk for milk or cream; low-fat yogurt for sour cream; cottage cheese for cream cheese.

Bake, broil, or roast on a rack so meat will remain above the drippings. Cool and remove the layer of fat from stews or soups.

Don't sample foods as you cook. If you can't resist, chew sugarless gum as you cook. Adjust seasoning by smell, not taste.

Keep carrot, celery, and cucumber sticks in the refrigerator at all times in case of snack attack. Keep your refrigerator on the "bare side" by throwing out leftovers and only buying what is needed for one week's menus.

Don't put bowls of nuts or candy around the house. Food should be confined to the kitchen.

LIFESTYLE TIPS

If you snack when you come home before dinner, either go for a walk, have dinner time moved up, come home later, or eat a few celery or carrot sticks.

Work off your emotions by exercising, not by eating. Call a friend and participate in a sport together—you'll find a friend a lot more comforting than a piece of cake. Just the act of calling may make the anger or depression leave, and exercise is a good tranquilizer.

If you drive to work or to shop, park farther away. A few extra steps each day add up over a year. Use the stairs rather than the escalator or elevator.

If you have to bend over to pick something up, bend over but leave it there, straighten up again, then bend over and pick it up. If you have to reach up on a shelf, follow the same strategy.

Carry things one item at a time. Take out the garbage one bag at a time. Don't shout messages to people, walk over to them. Don't ask the kids to do your little errands, do them yourself. In fact, be a volunteer for whatever needs to be done.

If you are brown-bagging, go for a walk around the block or through the building after lunch. Climb two flights of stairs during short breaks.

Stand some of the time you usually sit. Walk around a bit while talking on the telephone. Rise up and down on your toes. Wiggle your toes and fingers often while sitting.

Rearrange cabinets and drawers so that you have to reach more often or walk farther to them.

Start each day with positive thoughts. Be proud that you are dieting and will gain control, not pounds.

Get adequate sleep. Cut back on TV. If you must watch a show, exercise while watching it. Catch up on your hobbies, letter writing, repair work, sewing and phone calls to keep you busy *away* from food. Brush the dog. Trade chores with others to stay away from the refrigerator. Organize your closets and files, or take inventory of household articles for insurance purposes, or wash the car, but keep busy. You'll burn calories and keep away from the refrigerator.

Enter the house through a door that does not lead you to the kitchen. Stay out of the kitchen as much as you can. If you need a drink, get a glass of water from the upstairs bathroom. You need the exercise anyhow. And, above all, don't use the kitchen phone.

Don't add extra stresses. Don't try to diet at the same time you want to stop smoking, get married, move to a new house, or change jobs.

Take in your clothes as you lose weight. You'll look better and will have no spares to expand back into.

MISCELLANEOUS TIPS

One lady found pleasure in placing five one-pound plastic bags of lard in the refrigerator. Every time she lost a pound, she ceremoniously dropped a pound of lard in the garbage.

Tape pictures of yourself on the refrigerator. One picture should be your "before" picture and the other, one when you were at your best weight.

Establish a reward system for each subgoal reached. Don't use food as your reward, but treat yourself to a "little something nice"—a magazine, book, record, house plant, movie, play, trip to the beauty salon, day trip, jewelry or cosmetics. Women sometimes enjoy buying an article of clothing that is the next size smaller.

Every time you win a mental battle over food, reward yourself by putting money in a special bank. Use that money to splurge on YOU.

A reward system that has special value has been developed by Dr. Rick Guyton and is incorporated into the Slendernow Diet Program record system I'll discuss shortly.

HUNGER FIGHTING

Occasionally a little hunger sneaks up on us all, even when we're not dieting. But, learn to tell the difference between empty stomach *hunger* and boredom *appetite.*

Realize that hunger can be waited out. Daydream for a few minutes. Learn to convert that hunger sensation from a cue to eat to a feeling of success by telling yourself, "What great news, I am losing weight to become the person I wish to be." The hunger sensation is telling you more fat is being burned.

When you have a snack attack, first imagine yourself as fat as the refrigerator, and then, as you drink a glass of water and maybc eat a celery stick, imagine yourself at your desired weight. THINK THIN!

A few years ago, I reported how to use finger pressure to stop hunger pains. The technique, a form of acupressure, was developed by three physicians, Dr. Robert E. Williner of Miami, Dr. Keith Kenyon of Van Nuys, California, and Dr. Albert Fields of the State of California's Board of Medical Assurance.

One technique is to insert your index finger gently into both of your ears with your palms turned toward your face. Now bring your thumbs toward your index fingers until you find the little bump of cartilage at the front of your external ear, called the tragus. Gently squeeze the tragus (not the large lobes at the bottom of your ears) and firmly massage the tragus between your thumbs and index fingers for at least a minute.

As alternate technique is to place your index fingers in the small depressions immediately in front of your ear tragus, and then rub, with slight pressure, in a circular motion for at least a minute.

Now a German acupressure expert, Dr. Frank Bahr, has developed another effective technique, utilizing a pressure point between the center of your upper lip and nose. With your thumb inside your mouth under the lip at its center and your index finger on the outside of the mouth of the aforementioned spot, massage for a full minute with moderate pressure.

If you use either technique, your sensation of hunger will abate.

BEHAVIOR CHAINS

If you are concerned about analyzing your eating behavior, Dr. Rick Guyton points out that it is sometimes helpful to diagram *behavioral chains.* For all of us, eating is triggered by internal and/or external cues. If we are able to identify those cues, we may be successful in postponing or eliminating an eating episode. Examples of behavioral chains are given in Figure 13.1.

The obvious purpose in constructing behavioral chains is to identify the cues that triggered the eating episode. If the individual can recognize appropriate cues, future episodes might be postponed or prevented.

FIGURE 13.1

Behavioral chains help you to analyze your eating habits.

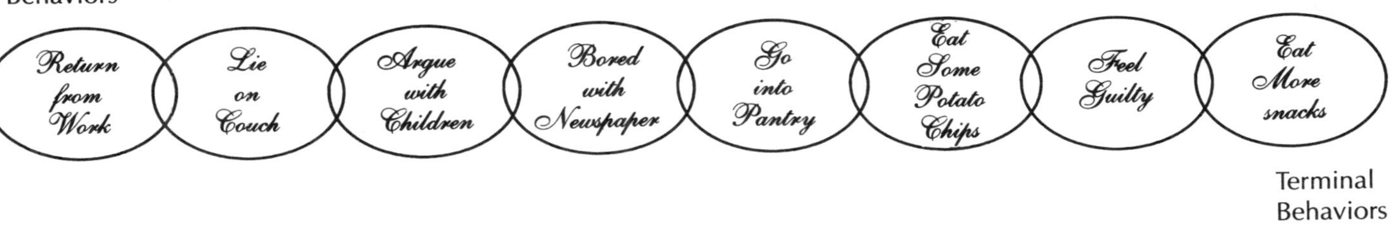

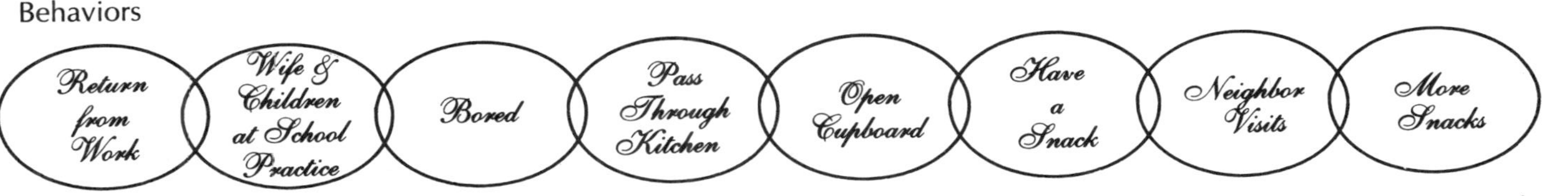

Reprinted from *Breaking the Eating Habit*, by permission of the copyright owner, Dr. Rick Guyton.

ACTIVITIES TO POSTPONE EATING EPISODES

Enjoyable Activities

softball

soccer

swimming

table tennis

work in flower beds

jogging

Work Activities

repair or wash auto.

paint home

vacuum carpet

clean out garage

rake leaves

make beds

When These Activities Should Be Utilized

wanted some cake—postponed desire by jogging

wanted a snack—washed auto

wanted coffee and roll—worked out with the neighbors

wanted crackers and cheese—read new book

wanted dessert after a meal—drank 2 glasses of water

If there are particular problems that arise where solutions are difficult to conceptualize, it is sometimes helpful to analyze the problem utilizing the *Special Problems Sheet*. Note the following sample.

SPECIAL PROBLEMS

Statement of the Problem: *I often snack in the evening between the hours of 8:00–9:30 just after dinner.*

Possible Solutions to the Problem:

(1) When I return home from job, immediately initiate some form of physical exercise.

(2) Have dinner later in the evening.

(3) Do not come home until the dinner hour.

(4) Drink a glass of water and eat 2 carrots when I have the desire to snack.

Best Solution and Future Plan of Action: *Put on jumpsuit and go jogging just prior to dinner, move the dinner hour back to 7:30, remove all snack foods from the house.*

Reward System and Consequence

Before beginning your behavioral change system, it is very important that you collaborate with a friend or relative and establish an adequate reward system to motivate you through this eight-week program. A monetary reward established with yourself is usually ideal, such as setting aside fifty dollars which will be yours if you successfully complete the project, but will be forfeited to your spouse or companion. Indeed, contractual rewards should be established for weekly as well as program-long success. The following forms and contracts should be scrupulously maintained throughout the program. Under no circumstances should food or alcohol be utilized in this reward system.

EIGHT-WEEK BEHAVIORAL CHANGE SYSTEM CONTRACT

I. ______________________________, will complete all
(Name)
eight weeks of the recommended program including tabulation of all significant data on specified forms, daily exercise, and preparation of meals to the No Flab diet plan.

II. Consequences provided by me:

A. If contract is kept ______________________________
(reward)
____

B. If contract is broken ______________________________

____

III. Consequence provided by others: (relative or friend)

A. If contract if kept ______________________________

____

B. If contract is broken ______________________________

____

Signed ______________________

Witness ______________________
(relative or friend)

Reprinted from *Breaking the Eating Habit,* by permission of the copyright owner, Dr. Rick Guyton.

FIRST WEEK *

Weekly Reward System

If I successfully complete all forms and work toward altering my eating behaviors throughout the week, my reward will be ______

____

____

____

____

____

It will be received on

(date) ______________

Signed ______________

Partner ______________

*Repeat this program using these charts as examples, for the full eight weeks.

EATING DIARY FOR (DAY OF WEEK) ______

DAILY BEHAVIORAL CHANGE PROJECT ______

	Duration of Eating Episode	Meal or Snack	Eating Location	Type and Amount of Food	Behavioral Project
7:00 a.m.					
9:00 a.m.					
1:00 p.m.					
5:00 p.m.					
9:00 p.m.					

EATING DIARY FOR (DAY OF WEEK) ____________________

DAILY BEHAVIORAL CHANGE PROJECT ____________________

	Duration of Eating Episode	Meal or Snack	Eating Location	Type and Amount of Food	Behavioral Project
7:00 a.m.					
9:00 a.m.					
1:00 p.m.					
5:00 p.m.					
9:00 p.m.					

EATING DIARY FOR (DAY OF WEEK) ____________________

DAILY BEHAVIORAL CHANGE PROJECT ____________________

	Duration of Eating Episode	Meal or Snack	Eating Location	Type and Amount of Food	Behavioral Project
7:00 a.m.					
9:00 a.m.					
1:00 p.m.					
5:00 p.m.					
9:00 p.m.					

EATING DIARY FOR (DAY OF WEEK) ______________________________

DAILY BEHAVIORAL CHANGE PROJECT ______________________________

	Duration of Eating Episode	Meal or Snack	Eating Location	Type and Amount of Food	Behavioral Project
7:00 a.m.					
9:00 a.m.					
1:00 p.m.					
5:00 p.m.					
9:00 p.m.					

EATING DIARY FOR (DAY OF WEEK) ______________________

DAILY BEHAVIORAL CHANGE PROJECT ______________________

	Duration of Eating Episode	Meal or Snack	Eating Location	Type and Amount of Food	Behavioral Project
7:00 a.m.					
9:00 a.m.					
1:00 p.m.					
5:00 p.m.					
9:00 p.m.					

EATING DIARY FOR (DAY OF WEEK) ______________________________

DAILY BEHAVIORAL CHANGE PROJECT ______________________________

	Duration of Eating Episode	Meal or Snack	Eating Location	Type and Amount of Food	Behavioral Project
7:00 a.m.					
9:00 a.m.					
1:00 p.m.					
5:00 p.m.					
9:00 p.m.					

EATING DIARY FOR (DAY OF WEEK) ______

DAILY BEHAVIORAL CHANGE PROJECT ______

	Duration of Eating Episode	Meal or Snack	Eating Location	Type and Amount of Food	Behavioral Project
7:00 a.m.					
9:00 a.m.					
1:00 p.m.					
5:00 p.m.					
9:00 p.m.					

Behavioral chains help you to analyze your eating habits.

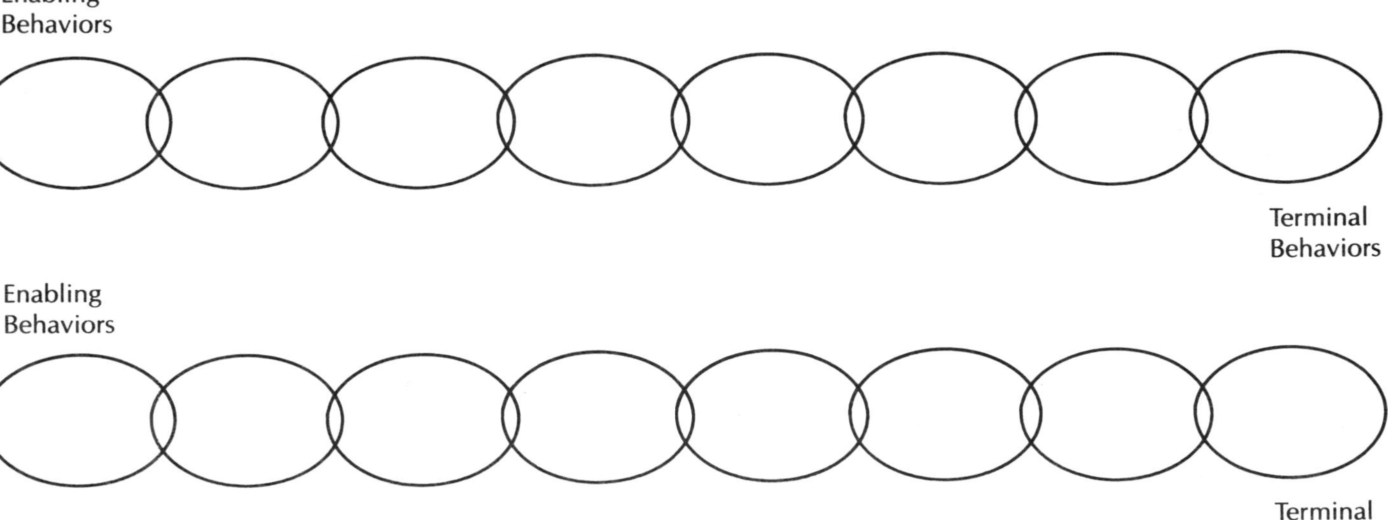

Reprinted from *Breaking the Eating Habit*, by permission of the copyright owner, Dr. Rick Guyton.

BEHAVIORAL INVENTORY

Item	S	M	T	W	T	F	S	TOTAL
No snack food in house								
Exercising daily								
No TV while eating								
Utensils down between bites								
Planning meals in advance								
Disposing of all leftovers								
Using smaller plates								
All foods in opaque containers								
Cooking only one serving								
Eating at specified place								
Introducing delays in meals								
Enjoying meals								
Counting calories								
Maintaining daily records								
Leaving food on plate								
Minimizing contact with food								
Using timer to delay snacks								
Had shake within 20 minutes after getting up								

_____ Week

_____ Weight at the start of the week

_____ Weight at the end of the week

_____ Weight loss for the week

Based on a format used by Dr. Rick Guyton in *Breaking the Eating Habit*. Reprinted with permission.

PRESCRIPTION SHEET FOR SPECIAL PROBLEMS

Statement of the Problem: ______________________________

____

____

____

Possible Solutions to the Problem: ______________________

____

____

____

Best Solution and Future Plan of Action: ________________

____

____

____

CONGRATULATIONS! You have just completed the first week of your Behavioral Change System.

1. Weigh yourself and plot your weight and measurements on Table 6.1 in Chapter 6.
2. Study the data you have collected by maintaining your eating diaries and completing the specialized forms for the past week.
3. Identify particular cues that triggered your eating episodes. Devise a plan of action for the next week which will help you eliminate those cues.
4. Consult with your partner in planning your program for the next week. Reinforce each other's commitment to complete the program.
5. Plan your meals for the next week according to the sample menus found in Chapter 10.

14

If you prefer to diet privately and quietly and have no trouble getting motivated, this chapter is not for you. However, if you need extra motivation and enjoy companionship, read on.

Friends with common goals encourage each other by lending the support of knowing that others share the problems.

Besides empathy and companionship, small neighborhood "clubs" can help keep you on schedule. Meetings are convenient to check your progress, but more importantly, they keep the program schedule in your thoughts.

You can either form your own club of two or three friends or join a larger permanent club that has experienced counselors. Formal clubs have proven to be effective in aiding people in moderating their eating and exercise lifestyle, as well as helping people break unhealthy habits.

Alcoholics Anonymous and various antismoking clubs have helped many, many people improve their lives. Some people will exercise regularly only when they belong to a health or exercise club. If you find it more interesting to do things with friends or just to get out, seriously consider forming your own club or joining an existing club.

FORMING YOUR GROUP

If you want to lose weight but really never seem to get around to it, try talking a friend or two into doing it with you. Nearly everyone needs to lose a few pounds and most need a little more encouragement to get started. Once you and your friends actually start, you will find that it is much easier than you think. A journey has to begin with a first step.

Now admittedly, you might injure some feelings if you approach friends out of the blue and suggest that they need to lose weight. But haven't your friends mentioned it themselves recently? If so, use that as an opening. You might suggest something like, "You know, I've been thinking about what you said about wanting to lose weight. I want to lose a few pounds also. Why don't we help each other? We can exercise together, swap menus, encourage each other, and keep each other on the right path. Maybe we can even make it fun." After two of you decide to work together, finding a third friend is easy.

However, don't sit around looking for a third friend. Start the Slendernow Diet together. After a week or so, you'll have lost several pounds and you'll feel better. Your friends will soon notice and will be asking to join the "club." As you each reach a subgoal, all will share the pride and enjoyment.

It is important that you meet once a week to measure your progress and solve any problems that may arise. You can exercise all together four times a week or at every other exercise session, if you wish.

Some people have done this and felt so good about it that they have continued to help others diet successfully even after they have reached their own desired weight.

FORMAL CLUBS

A number of individuals who were helped by earlier versions of the Slendernow Diet Program were so enthusiastic about their results that they formed neighborhood clubs to help others. They have formed the "Slendernow Neighborhood Clubs of America."

(I have no financial or any other connection with this group other than the fact that they helped test the Slendernow Diet Program for me. Their suggestions, comments, and even recipes were quite helpful in perfecting the Slendernow Diet.)

I don't know if there is a Slendernow Neighborhood Club of America near you, but you can find out by writing to:

Futuron Industries
Slendernow Neighborhood Clubs of America
4419 Westgrove
Dallas, Texas 75248

The results achieved by such clubs are not only good for the dieters, but they are good for the souls of the club directors. The following letter from Carol Koester of Orlando, Florida, illustrates this point.

> As a Slendernow Neighborhood Clubs of America director, I have seen many people helped, not only with weight problems, but with improved health and lasting lifestyles as well.
>
> One case in particular was a 21-year-old woman who had suddenly gone from being underweight at 18 to 80 pounds overweight. She had dropped out of college and become almost completely reclusive, with a phobia of crowds. Her family were all slim and didn't understand her problems at all. She had gone from one expensive weight-loss program to another, with no good results, even trying drugs, under a physician's direction. The only things she lost were her hair, her health, and her outgoing personality!
>
> When she joined the Slendernow Neighborhood Clubs of America, her weight loss was slow but steady—about 2 to 3 pounds a week. But her personality change was miraculous. The behavior modification course, together with the personal caring and understanding on the part of all the members, helped her overcome her phobias, and she was able to return to dorm life in a distant college after 6 months.

If you enjoy helping others, after you've been helped by the Slendernow Diet Program, consider starting your own Slendernow Neighborhood Diet Club.

15

Human nature is such that once someone has achieved his weight goal, he asumes that he will keep trim. "Boy, I'll never let myself get fat again. It's more fun not to diet." Ah, eternal optimism! However, unless new eating habits have been learned, history is doomed to repeat itself.

If you have made lifestyle changes discussed in Chapter 13, you *will* maintain your desired weight. However, you may have questions about how to switch from a reducing diet to a nonfattening, nondieting regimen. This chapter discusses the transition period and how to plan sensible eating habits that will maintain *your* desired weight.

The prescription is simple: if you regulate your food intake at the proper level to maintain your desired weight for a few weeks, your body will reset its regulatory mechanism to automatically maintain your desired weight.

The four-week post-diet program is not very elaborate, but it is just enough of a reminder to keep you tuned in to a better lifestyle. You should continue to keep a food notebook, and a record of daily weight and exercise.

You will need to keep your calorie intake in line with your calorie needs for your weight. If you exceed this need, you will gain weight again. An important difference between reducing and maintaining, of course, is the quantity of food permitted, but another difference is that during your maintenance program you do not have to worry about your daily calorie intake as much as when you are reducing, but instead you can relax a little and concentrate on your *average* calorie intake. In everyday living in the real world, wc sometimes eat a little too much one day and then compensate for that by eating a little less the next day.

Your food notebook will help you keep track of your average daily calorie intake. It is critical to your long-term success to firmly establish your proper average daily calorie intake immediately. This will reset your appetite control mechanism, and from then on, you won't have to worry about calories. Your body will take proper care of calorie counting.

WEIGHT STABILIZATION AND DIET TRANSITION

When you reach your desired weight, you can begin to change over to your maintenance diet. You should change over gradually for two reasons. First of all, you actually want to fall one or two pounds below your desired weight to allow for "overshoot" error when you begin to stabilize. Secondly, a gradual changeover gives you better control of your weight and appetite.

The first step in the transition is to replace the second Diet Shake of the day with another meal. Not another main meal—that's too many calories—but a regular meal. Now you should be eating a Diet Shake for breakfast, an ordinary sensible lunch and a main-meal dinner. Of course, you can switch the lunch and dinner around if you prefer a larger meal at noon.

If you follow the one-milkshake-plus-two-meals-a-day plan for two weeks, you should lose the extra pound or two while adjusting to eating more food.

However, if during this period your weight goes up over your desired weight, immediately return to the basic two Diet Shakes Slendernow Diet until you are back to your desired weight. (Women can allow for water retention during the monthly cycle.)

When you have brought your weight back down, resume your one Diet Shake plus two meals a day, but eat fewer calories in your meals.

After two weeks of not exceeding your desired weight, proceed to Step 2 of the Slendernow Diet Maintenance Plan.

In Step 2, you should have a regular breakfast every other day, alternating with a Diet Shake. Your weight should stabilize during this period, but if at any time it exceeds your desired weight, immediately go back to the regular Slendernow Diet Program. When you drop below your desired weight again, go on the one-Diet-Shake-a-day-plus-two-meals plan of Step 1 for three days and then start Step 2 again, but watch your calorie intake more closely.

The secret is to *never* let your weight go above your desired weight again. I repeat! *Never again!* If it does, immediately switch to the Slendernow Diet. It is *much* easier to correct one pound than 5 or 10!

Some people choose to stay at Step 1. They enjoy a Diet Shake more than usual breakfast fare, and they feel it is better nourishment for them. When not dieting, they can add more fruits and flavorings.

The Diet Shake breakfast is great nutrition, especially for elderly people who don't wish to prepare elaborate breakfasts. It is also less expensive.

Adults of all ages will also find that a Diet Shake is better nutrition than junk-food snacks that they might be tempted to eat.

REGULAR MEALS

Calories are only part of the maintenance picture. Food quality and meal timing are as important as food quantity. Proper nourishment is important to your long-term health, and control of your blood insulin level is the important factor in determining how much fat you will store in your body.

Consider calories as money. You always ask yourself what you get for your money. Now ask yourself, what nourishment do you get for your allotted calories? The key is to eat only foods that are packed with nutrients, and leave foods alone that are "empty" calorie foods. "Empty" means that although there are many calories in the food, there are virtually no vitamins and minerals. Examples of empty calorie foods are candy, cakes, cookies, and others made with sugar and white flour. This doesn't mean that you can't ever enjoy sweets again, it merely means that you should satisfy your nutrient needs first, and only if you have room for more calories should you add sweets in moderation. You will find that unless you are very active, you will have little room for empty-calorie foods.

You don't have to be a nutritionist to learn to eat properly.

But you should know the basic four food groups and choose one from each per meal as suggested by the National Dairy Council.

Milk Group

1 cup milk
1 cup yogurt
1½ slices cheese
2 cups cottage cheese*

Meat Group

2 oz. cooked lean meat, fish, poultry
2 eggs
2 slices (2 oz.) cheese
½ cup cottage cheese*
1 cup dried beans, peas
4 tbsp. peanut butter

Fruit-Vegetable Group

½ cup juice
½ cup cooked
1 cup raw

(Commonly served portion such as medium-size apple or banana)

Grain (whole grain) Group

1 slice bread, whole wheat or rye
1 cup ready-to-eat cereal, unsweetened
½ cup cooked cereal, pasta, grits.

(*Count cheese as serving of milk OR meat, not both simultaneously)

How Many Calories

We have established what kinds of foods to eat and in what balance. Now let's determine how many calories *you* need.

The Food and Nutrition Board of the National Academy of Sciences has made approximations of energy needs for various groups of people.

The recommendations for adequate energy represent the average needs of people in each category, whereas for other nutrients, recommended intakes are high enough to meet the upper limits of variability of almost all people of this age and sex. A large number of individuals in the United States population are overweight and may require less energy than is recommended because they have sedentary work and leisure patterns. For individuals who are already obese, energy intake should be reduced below the suggested levels as but one of several measures in a sound program of weight control that includes increased exercise. However, adults or children who tend to gain excessive amounts of body fat while habitually consuming energy apparently appropriate to their body weight, sex, age, and activity should increase their physical activity until the desired weight is achieved. There are persuasive reasons for this view:

(1) Adequate energy intake is a requirement for efficient utilization of dietary protein for growth and maintenance.

(2) Many of the essential nutrients, particularly the minerals, are distributed widely and in low concentration in foods, especially in the low-cost staple commodities. It is therefore difficult to assure nutritional adequacy of diets that are low in energy content (less than 1800–2000 cal) unless fats, sugar, and alcohol are more rigidly restricted than is customary in most American households.

(3) There is evidence that a sedentary life contributes to degenerative arterial disease as well as to obesity and its many complications, notably diabetes mellitus and gallstones.

It should be emphasized that the maintenance of desirable body weight throughout adult life by an individual is dependent on achieving a balance between energy intake and energy output.

Allowances are specified for three age categories of average adults performing light activity. The age groups are 23 to 50 years, 51 to 75, and over 75 years (see Table 15.1).

TABLE 15.1

Average Daily Calorie Needs As Estimated by the National Research Council (1980 RDA)

CALORIE NEEDS FOR WOMEN			CALORIE NEEDS FOR MEN		
AGE (YEARS)	WEIGHT (POUNDS)	CALORIES	AGE (YEARS)	WEIGHT (POUNDS)	CALORIES
15–18	120	2100	15–18	145	2800
19–22	120	2100	19–22	154	2900
23–50	120	2000	23–50	154	2700
51–75	120	1800	51–75	154	2400
76+	120	1600	76+	154	2050

However, you are unique, an individual who is biochemically slightly different from the average. The Food and Nutrition Board sheds some light on adjusting the tables to better reflect your individual needs.

In the United States, people are presumed to live in an environment with a mean temperature of 20°C. and to wear clothing compatible with thermal comfort. Adjustments of the recommended average allowances must be made for increased physical activity, for body size, and, rarely, for climate. Adjustments must also be made for the special energy demands of pregnancy and lactation.

ACTIVITY

The dominant factor leading to variability in energy needs is the proportion of time an individual devotes to moderate and heavy activities in contrast with light or sedentary activities. The physical activity of people in the United States is generally considered to be light to sedentary.

For those in occupations entailing heavy work, energy allowances must be higher, especially if the individual does not reduce his recreational level of energy expenditure. A person whose occupation is quite sedentary may be active outside his employment and so have proportionately higher needs for energy. For this reason, it is not practical to express energy allowances according to occupational categories. The entire waking period should be considered in making adjustments and substituting different time spans for the activity categories.

In practice, the daily energy needs of a moderately active person of either sex and reference body weight might be increased by about 300 calories. For very active persons, such as athletes or military recruits in heavy training, miners, and heavy construction workers, the allowance may be considerably increased, according to the degree of exertion. In general, the adult energy requirement for maintenance with moderate activity is about 1.7 times the basal-energy expenditure for men and about 1.6 times basal for young women.

BODY SIZE

Persons of larger (or smaller) body size require proportionately more (or less) total energy per unit of time for activities, such as walking, that involve moving mass over distance. Their hourly resting metabolic rate will also be slightly higher or lower than the average. Energy allowances must be adjusted for the variations in requirements that result from these differences in body size.

Weight may be used as a basis for adapting allowances for differences in size within a given age-sex category, provided that the individuals are not appreciably over or under their desirable weight. Persons who are overweight often compensate for the increased energy cost of carrying their extra weight by decreasing daily activity. The true energy requirements of people who are underweight may be underestimated unless their desirable weight rather than their actual weight is used as the basis for estimating their energy allowances.

For the usual sedentary and moderately active groups, energy needs of about 70 percent of the adult population fall within a variation of ±400 calories. Adjustment for body size will need to be higher in persons who are both large and active.

AGE

Energy requirements decline gradually after early adulthood because the resting metabolic rate declines and physical activity may also be curtailed. Although the approximate rate of decline of the resting metabolism is known to be about 2 percent per decade in adults, it is difficult to estimate the degree of reduction in physical activity that is associated with advancing age. Men in occupations requiring light activity were found to have fairly constant activity patterns between ages 20 and 45; activity was less by about 200 calories/day in the years between ages 45 and 75 and by 500 calories/day after age 75.

It is proposed that energy allowances for persons between 51 and 75 years of age be reduced to about 90 percent of the amount required as a young adult, and for persons beyond age 75 years to about 75–80 percent of that amount. With advancing age, the differences in energy expenditure among individuals become more marked. (From *Recommended Dietary Allowances,* Ninth Edition 1980, The National Academy of Sciences, Washington, D.C.)

Another scale (Table 15.2) was formerly used by the Food and Nutrition Board. They seem to have abandoned that table in favor of the figures shown in Table 15.1. But I feel that Table 15.2 is still valid for healthy, active people, and it helps you to better zero in on your calorie needs.

You can only establish the proper balance for *you* by trial and response. Use the guidelines presented here as starting points. Make the changes to regular meals gradually, but if ever you should overshoot your desired weight, *immediately* revert to the Slendernow Diet.

Keep your food notebook for four weeks after you have finished the Slendernow Diet 8-week program so that you can calculate your equilibrium calories. Weigh yourself daily and exercise regularly. It's also a good idea to continue your vitamin and mineral pills to insure balanced nutrition.

It's actually easier to stabilize at your desired weight than to balance your checkbook.

TABLE 15.2

Calories Needed to Maintain Weight in Healthy, Active Persons (estimated by National Research Council, in RDA publication before 1980)

Weight	CALORIE NEEDS AT AGE 22	45	65
WOMEN			
88	1,550	1,450	1,300
99	1,700	1,550	1,450
110	1,800	1,650	1,500
121	1,950	1,800	1,650
128	2,000	1,850	1,700
132	2,050	1,900	1,700
143	2,200	2,000	1,850
154	2,300	2,100	1,950
MEN			
110	2,200	2,000	1,850
121	2,350	2,150	1,950
132	2,500	2,300	2,100
143	2,650	2,400	2,200
154	2,800	2,600	2,400
165	2,950	2,700	2,500
176	3,050	2,800	2,600
187	3,200	2,950	2,700
198	3,350	3,100	2,800
209	3,500	3,200	2,900
220	3,700	3,400	3,100

16

I receive many letters from hypoglycemics (people with low blood sugar) who are happy to have finally found a diet that they can use. It's hard enough to diet, but when your blood sugar level is prone to frequently dipping below the comfort level, dieting is next to impossible.

The Slendernow Diet is ideal for hypoglycemics and has helped many diabetics. I repeat: check with your physician before you start a diet, especially if you're a diabetic or hypoglycemic.

The secret for controlling both hypoglycemia and diabetes is to avoid overloading the blood with "food energy." Food energy is the glucose (blood sugar) formed from food as the digestive components enter the blood. When blood sugar increases rapidly, more insulin is required to remove the glucose from the blood, otherwise coma will result. Insulin opens cell membranes so that glucose enters the cells and is either burned for energy or converted to fat. Usually hypoglycemics and diabetics are very efficient at converting food energy into body fat.

The diabetic has trouble releasing enough insulin to keep the blood sugar level under control. Therefore, the diabetic doesn't want a large shot of glucose entering the blood.

Neither does the hypoglycemic. Although the hypoglycemic has adequate insulin to remove the blood sugar, the insulin must flood the bloodstream as a surge to prevent the blood sugar from rising. The effect is that of overkill.

It's much like trying to water a flower garden with a fireman's 2½-inch hose rather than with a ½-inch garden hose. By the time you turn it on, you have too much water and damage is done to the flowers.

In the case of the flood of insulin, so much blood sugar enters the cells that the blood sugar level drops into the discomfort zone and the person becomes irritable, shaky, weak, emotional, and hungry.

The question then becomes, "How does one prevent the rapid surge of blood sugar?" The answer is to avoid simple carbohydrates.

Simple carbohydrates, such as sugar, digest rapidly. Since they are simple molecules, digestive enzymes have little to do in preparing them for transport into the bloodstream. As a result, the entire calorie content of a simple carbohydrate enters into the blood almost all at once. It's as if one is given a shot of glucose with a hypodermic needle directly into the blood. Complex carbohydrates, proteins, and fats are more complicated molecules and require more digestive steps. As a result, they do not all digest at the same time and are not ready to enter the bloodstream all at once. They raise the blood sugar level at a slow rate and in an orderly manner. A flood of insulin is not required. If extra insulin needs to be released, it should come as only a trickle.

Thus, a low insulin-secreting diet is best for diabetics and hypoglycemics. If less insulin is in the bloodstream, less blood sugar is converted to stored fat.

The best way to prevent high insulin release is to avoid sugar as much as possible and to eat small meals. Several such meals are easier on the body and minimize the need for insulin.

The Slendernow Diet can be modified to meet the special needs of the hypoglycemic and diabetic. The Diet Shakes can be divided in half to provide smaller meals plus "snacks" at midmorning and midafternoon to maintain optimal blood sugar levels.

17

Someone once said that you can't lose weight by talking about it—you have to keep your mouth shut. Not quite true! You can easily lose weight while eating delicious milkshakes and tasty meals—but you cannot lose weight just by reading about it. Being overweight can only be corrected by you.

My job is done. Now it is up to you.

Will you be up to the task? Of course you will!

Let's sum up. You know the Slendernow Diet works! You know the Slendernow Diet is medically approved! You know the Slendernow Diet is nutritionally sound! You know the Slendernow Diet makes sense to you! You know the menus sound good; you always liked milkshakes anyway! You know there is no calorie counting or weighing of food! You know you should start!

If you put it off, you will continue putting it on! If you don't control your weight, your weight controls you. You may not know how you got overweight or may not have worried about it before, thinking that everyone "gets a little paunchy at my age." But that spare tire around your waist will be the most expensive one you can buy. Develop a sound body—not a round body.

Start with the three-day warmup plan. Take your measurements and mark your progress. Even though you may lose your targeted weight in one to four weeks, stay on the Slendernow Diet Program for eight weeks to insure that your new lifestyle habits become lifelong, long-life habits. They will add years to your life and life to your years.

Don't make excuses, "If I had time . . . if I could only get started. . . . if conditions were only different . . . if I were only younger . . ." DO IT NOW! It will be harder to do it later, and think of the fun you will miss if you wait. If you don't improve yourself now, you actually have made a decision to slip further into decline.

You control your destiny. You will regain your self-respect and increase the admiration others have in you. Don't allow bad habits or other people to control your eating habits.

Football coach Vince Lombardi said that the quality of a person's life is directly proportional to his commitment to excellence. Make that commitment. You can become better and better with each day, each week, each month, each year. Your own self-image is at stake and that is your most important possession. After you like yourself again, the world will look much better to you.

Give the Slendernow Diet a chance and it will give you a healthier, trimmer body. You owe it to yourself and your loved ones—and they'll love you all the more.

DO IT!

APPENDIX

Content of protein, carbohydrate and fat, and average caloric values of some common foods.

FOOD	AVERAGE SERVING (G)	PROTEIN (G)	CARBOHYDRATE (G)	FAT (G)	TOTAL CAL PER SERVING
FRUITS					
Apple	100	0.4	14.2	0.5	65
Grapefruit	100	0.6	12.2	0.1	50
Orange	100	0.8	11.6	0.2	50
Strawberries	100	1.0	7.4	0.6	40
VEGETABLES					
Asparagus	50	0.9	1.6	0.1	10
Beans, baked	100	6.9	9.6	2.5	130
Beans, green	100	2.3	7.4	0.3	40
Beans, lima, green	100	7.5	23.5	0.8	130
Brussels sprouts	100	4.2	8.0	0.5	55
Cabbage	30	0.5	1.7	0.1	10
Celery	50	0.6	1.7	0.05	10
Corn	100	3.7	20.5	1.2	110
Cucumber	60	0.5	1.9	0.1	10

Lettuce	50	0.6	1.5	0.2	10
Onions	10	0.2	1.0	0.03	5
Peas, green	100	7.0	17.0	0.5	100
Potatoes, sweet	100	1.8	27.4	0.7	125
Potatoes, white	150	3.3	27.6	0.2	125
Radish	35	0.5	2.0	0.04	10
CEREALS					
Bread, white (1 sl)	30	2.8	15.9	0.4	80
Bread, whole wheat	30	2.9	14.9	0.3	75
Macaroni	25	3.4	18.5	0.1	90
Oatmeal	25	4.0	16.9	0.2	100
NUTS					
Almonds	15	3.2	2.6	8.2	100
Brazil nuts	15	2.6	1.1	10.0	105
Coconut, dry	15	0.9	4.7	8.6	100
Peanuts	15	3.9	3.7	5.8	80
Pecans	15	1.7	2.0	10.7	85

Content of protein, carbohydrate and fat, and average caloric values of some common foods.

FOOD	AVERAGE SERVING (G)	PROTEIN (G)	CARBOHYDRATE (G)	FAT (G)	TOTAL CAL PER SERVING
MEATS & POULTRY PRODUCTS					
Bacon	30	3.2	—	19.4	190
Beef, liver	100	20.4	2.5	16.3	150
Beef, steak	100	18.9	—	18.5	240
Chicken	100	21.5	—	2.5	110
Duck	100	18.0	—	19.0	245
Eggs, two	100	13.4	—	10.5	150
Fish, cod	100	11.1	—	0.2	45
Fish, sardines in oil	100	19.2	—	25.5	315
Fish, white	100	22.9	—	6.5	150
Ham	100	19.8	—	20.8	265
Pork, chops	75	12.5	—	22.6	255
Pork, sausage	75	9.8	—	33.1	300
Veal, cutlet	100	17.8	1.5	16.0	220
DAIRY PRODUCTS					
Butter	10	0.06	—	8.2	75
Cheese, American	25	7.2	0.08	9.0	110

Cream, sweet	15	0.4	0.7	2.8	30
Ice cream	100	4.0	20.0	14.0	220
Milk, skim	250	8.5	12.8	0.8	95
Milk, whole	250	8.3	12.5	10.0	170
MISCELLANEOUS					
Apple pie	200	3.2	64.0	18.2	430
Marmalade, orange	10	0.06	8.5	0.01	35
Sponge cake	100	11.8	62.0	7.5	360
Sugar, 1 tsp.	5	—	5.0	—	20

Index